Molecular Imaging of Prostate Cancer

Guest Editor

HOSSEIN JADVAR, MD, PhD, MPH, MBA

PET CLINICS

www.pet.theclinics.com

Consulting Editor
ABASS ALAVI, MD,
MD (Hon), PhD (Hon), DSc (Hon)

April 2009 • Volume 4 • Number 2

SAUNDERS an imprint of ELSEVIER, Inc.

W.B. SAUNDERS COMPANY
A Division of Elsevier Inc.

1600 John F. Kennedy Boulevard ● Suite 1800 ● Philadelphia, Pennsylvania 19103-2899

http://www.theclinics.com

PET CLINICS Volume 4, Number 2
April 2009 ISSN 1556-8598, ISBN 10: 1-4377-0880-3, ISBN-13: 978-1-4377-0880-6

Editor: Barton Dudlick
Developmental Editor: Theresa Collier

PET Clinics (ISSN 1556-8598) is published quarterly by Elsevier Inc., 360 Park Avenue South, New York, NY 10010-1710. Months of issue are January, April, July, and October. Periodicals postage paid at New York, NY, and additional mailing offices. Subscription prices per year are $196.00 (US individuals), $274.00 (US institutions), $97.00 (US students), $223.00 (Canadian individuals), $306.00 (Canadian institutions), $118.00 (Canadian students), $237.00 (foreign individuals), $306.00 (foreign institutions), and $118.00 (foreign students). To receive student and resident rate, orders must be accompanied by name of affiliated institution, date of term, and the signature of program/residency coordinator on institution letterhead. Orders will be billed at individual rate until proof of status is received. Foreign air speed delivery is included in all Clinics subscription prices. All prices are subject to change without notice. POSTMASTER: Send address changes to PET Clinics, Elsevier Health Sciences Division, Subscription Customer Service, 3251 Riverport Lane, Maryland Heights, MO 63043. **Customer service: 1-800-654-2452 (US and Canada). From outside of the US and Canada, call 314-447-8871. Fax: 314-417-8029. E-mail: JournalsCustomerService-usa@elsevier.com (for print support); JournalsOnlineSupport-usa@elsevier.com (for online support).**

Reprints. For copies of 100 or more of articles in this publication, please contact the Commercial Reprints Department, Elsevier Inc., 360 Park Avenue South, New York, NY 10010-1710. Tel.: 212-633-3812; Fax: 212-462-1935; E-mail: reprints@elsevier.com.

Printed and bound in the United Kingdom
Transferred to Digital Print 2011

Contributors

CONSULTING EDITOR

ABASS ALAVI, MD,
MD (Hon), PhD (Hon), DSc (Hon)
Professor of Radiology, Department of Radiology,
Division of Nuclear Medicine, Hospital of
University of Pennsylvania, University of
Pennsylvania School of Medicine, Philadelphia,
Pennsylvania

GUEST EDITOR

HOSSEIN JADVAR, MD, PhD, MPH, MBA
Associate Professor of Radiology and Biomedical
Engineering, Director of Radiology Research,
Keck School of Medicine, University of Southern
California, Los Angeles, California

AUTHORS

ABASS ALAVI, MD,
MD (Hon), PhD (Hon), DSc (Hon)
Professor of Radiology, Department of Radiology,
Division of Nuclear Medicine, Hospital of
University of Pennsylvania, University of
Pennsylvania School of Medicine, Philadelphia,
Pennsylvania

MARTIN S. ALLEN-AUERBACH, MD
Assistant Professor, Department of Molecular and
Medical Pharmacology, Division of Ahmanson
Biological Imaging, David Geffen School of
Medicine, University of California Los Angeles, Los
Angeles, California

MOHSEN BEHESHTI, MD, FEBNM, FASNC
Associate Professor of Nuclear Medicine and
Senior Attending Physician, Department
of Nuclear Medicine and Endocrinology, PET-CT
Center Linz, St. Vincent's Hospital, Linz, Austria

MATTHIAS R. BENZ, MD
Research Fellow, Department of Molecular and
Medical Pharmacology, Division of Ahmanson
Biological Imaging, David Geffen School of
Medicine, University of California Los Angeles, Los
Angeles, California

JOHANNES CZERNIN, MD
Professor, Department of Molecular and Medical
Pharmacology, Division of Ahmanson Biological
Imaging, David Geffen School of Medicine,
University of California Los Angeles, Los Angeles,
California

EKTA GUPTA, MD
Department of Radiology, Hospital of the
University of Pennsylvania, University of
Pennsylvania School of Medicine, Philadelphia,
Pennsylvania

HOSSEIN JADVAR, MD, PhD, MPH, MBA
Associate Professor of Radiology and Biomedical
Engineering, Director of Radiology Research,
Keck School of Medicine, University of Southern
California, Los Angeles, California

WERNER LANGSTEGER, MD, FACE
Professor of Nuclear Medicine and Chief,
Department of Nuclear Medicine and
Endocrinology, PET-CT Center Linz, St. Vincent's
Hospital, Linz, Austria

ALEXANDER LIN, MD
Assistant Professor, Department of Radiation
Oncology, Hospital of the University of
Pennsylvania, University of Pennsylvania School
of Medicine, Philadelphia, Pennsylvania

HOMER A. MACAPINLAC, MD
Professor and Chairman, Department of Nuclear
Medicine, University of Texas M. D. Anderson
Cancer Center, Houston, Texas

ERIC M. ROHREN, MD, PhD
Associate Professor, Department of Nuclear
Medicine, University of Texas M. D. Anderson
Cancer Center, Houston, Texas

DREW A. TORIGIAN, MD, MA
Department of Radiology, Hospital of the
University of Pennsylvania, University
of Pennsylvania School of Medicine, Philadelphia,
Pennsylvania

NEHA VAPIWALA, MD
Assistant Professor, Department of Radiation
Oncology, Hospital of the University of
Pennsylvania, University of Pennsylvania School
of Medicine, Philadelphia, Pennsylvania

Contents

Although PET using fludeoxyglucose F 18 (FDG) is a promising modality for metabolic imaging of different tumors, the results in prostate cancer have been somewhat inconsistent. Low FDG avidity of most prostate cancer cells and urinary activity are suggested as the main limitations of FDG PET for the evaluation of prostate cancer. Prostate cancer exhibits increased choline metabolism, which is the rationale for using radiolabeled choline for PET. This article describes the basic concepts of radiolabeled choline regarding pharmacokinetics, radiation dosimetry, synthesis, and biodistribution, in addition to advances concerning clinical PET using 11C- and 18F-choline in primary staging and restaging of prostate cancer patients.

There are significant limitations in the current options for imaging of patients with prostate carcinoma. Although fluorodeoxyglucose is the mainstay of clinical imaging, many other isotope and tracer combinations can be imaged with PET. One of the strengths of nuclear imaging lies in the variety of radiotracers capable of being imaged. In the last 15 years, various compounds have been studied in the hope of identifying the ideal imaging agent for prostate cancer. In this article, the use of imaging agents other than fluorodeoxyglucose, choline, and acetate is discussed.

PET imaging has become an integral component of the diagnosis and management of a substantial number of lymphatic and solid malignancies. One of the greatest dilemmas in prostate cancer remains the need for greater personalization of treatment recommendations based on the true extent of disease, so that patients with extraprostatic, micrometastatic disease can be identified early and managed accordingly. These sites currently remain under the level of detection with standard imaging and continue to confound clinicians. Novel PET tracers to complement anatomic data from CT and MR imaging can truly make a difference, and ongoing research holds the greatest promise.

PET Clinics

THE CLINICS ARE NOW AVAILABLE ONLINE!

Access your subscription at:
www.theclinics.com

GOAL STATEMENT

The goal of the *PET Clinics* is to keep practicing radiologists and radiology residents up to date with current clinical practice in positron emission tomography by providing timely articles reviewing the state of the art in patient care.

ACCREDITATION

PET Clinics is planned and implemented in accordance with the Essential Areas and Policies of the Accreditation Council for Continuing Medical Education (ACCME) through the joint sponsorship of the University of Virginia School of Medicine and Elsevier. The University of Virginia School of Medicine is accredited by the ACCME to provide continuing medical education for physicians.

The University of Virginia School of Medicine designates this educational activity for a maximum of 15 AMA PRA Category 1 Credits™ for each issue, 60 credits per year. Physicians should only claim credit commensurate with the extent of their participation in the activity.

The American Medical Association has determined that physicians not licensed in the US who participate in this CME activity are eligible for a maximum of 15 AMA PRA Category 1 Credits™ for each issue, 60 credits per year.

Category 1 credit can be earned by reading the text material, taking the CME examination online at http://www.theclinics.com/home/cme, and completing the evaluation. After taking the test, you will be required to review any and all incorrect answers. Following completion of the test and evaluation, your credit will be awarded and you may print your certificate.

FACULTY DISCLOSURE/CONFLICT OF INTEREST

The University of Virginia School of Medicine, as an ACCME accredited provider, endorses and strives to comply with the Accreditation Council for Continuing Medical Education (ACCME) Standards of Commercial Support, Commonwealth of Virginia statutes, University of Virginia policies and procedures, and associated federal and private regulations and guidelines on the need for disclosure and monitoring of proprietary and financial interests that may affect the scientific integrity and balance of content delivered in continuing medical education activities under our auspices.

The University of Virginia School of Medicine requires that all CME activities accredited through this institution be developed independently and be scientifically rigorous, balanced and objective in the presentation/discussion of its content, theories and practices.

All authors/editors participating in an accredited CME activity are expected to disclose to the readers relevant financial relationships with commercial entities occurring within the past 12 months (such as grants or research support, employee, consultant, stock holder, member of speakers bureau, etc.). The University of Virginia School of Medicine will employ appropriate mechanisms to resolve potential conflicts of interest to maintain the standards of fair and balanced education to the reader. Questions about specific strategies can be directed to the Office of Continuing Medical Education, University of Virginia School of Medicine, Charlottesville, Virginia.

The faculty and staff of the University of Virginia Office of Continuing Medical Education have no financial affiliations to disclose.

The authors/editors listed below have identified no professional or financial affiliations for themselves or their spouse/partner:
Abass Alavi, MD, MD(Hon), PhD(Hon), DSc(Hon) (Consulting Editor); Martin S. Allen-Auerbach, MD; Mohsen Beheshti, MD, FEBNM, FASNC; Matthias R. Benz, MD; Barton Dudlick (Acquisitions Editor); Ekta Gupta, MD; Hossein Jadvar, MD, PhD, MPH, MBA (Guest Editor); Werner Langsteger, MD, FACE; Alexander Lin, MD; Patrice Rehm, MD (Test Author); Eric M. Rohren, MD, PhD; Drew A. Torigian, MD, MA; and Neha Vapiwala, MD.

The authors/editors listed below identified the following professional or financial affiliations for themselves or their spouse/partner:
Johannes Czernin, MD is a consultant for Siemens.
Homer A. Macapinlac, MD serves on the Speakers Bureau for Siemens Medical Solutions, Inc., GE Healthcare, Cardinal Health, and International Atomic Energy Agency, serves on the Advisory Committee for GE Healthcare and International Atomic Energy Agency, and is a consultant for International Atomic Energy Agency.

Disclosure of Discussion of Non-FDA Approved Uses for Pharmaceutical Products and/or Medical Devices.
The University of Virginia School of Medicine, as an ACCME provider, requires that all faculty presenters identify and disclose any off-label uses for pharmaceutical and medical device products. The University of Virginia School of Medicine recommends that each physician fully review all the available data on new products or procedures prior to clinical use.

TO ENROLL

To enroll in the PET Clinics Continuing Medical Education program, call customer service at 1-800-654-2452 or visit us online at www.theclinics.com/home/cme. The CME program is available to subscribers for an additional fee of $175.00.

Preface

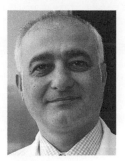

Hossein Jadvar, MD, PhD, MPH, MBA
Guest Editor

Prostate cancer continues to be a major public health problem. The incidence of prostate cancer is expected to rise as longevity increases. Imaging of prostate cancer is particularly challenging because of the biological and clinical heterogeneity of the disease. Although PET with [F-18]-fluorodeoxyglucose (FDG) has found important diagnostic and, to some extent, prognostic utility in many cancers, the situation for prostate cancer remains uncertain and controversial. The recent National Oncologic PET Registry data suggest that there may be a role for FDG-PET in prostate cancer. PET is usually and unjustly synonymous with FDG-PET. In fact, there are almost an unlimited number of radiotracers that may be designed for PET imaging interrogation of various disease processes, including cancer.

In this issue of *PET Clinics*, we have focused on prostate cancer. An overview of the role of imaging in prostate cancer is presented in the first article. In the second article, Drs. Gupta and Torigian from the University of Pennsylvania, describe the role of MRI in prostate cancer, which is commonly used for the evaluation of the prostate gland for primary cancer or other conditions because PET has a limited role in the initial diagnosis and staging of primary prostate cancer. In the third article, the potential role of FDG, the most common PET radiotracer, is summarized. The next two articles discuss the potential and emerging roles of radiolabeled acetate and choline in the imaging evaluation of prostate cancer, respectively. The acetate article is presented by Dr. Czernin and his group at UCLA, and the choline article is presented by an experienced group from St. Vincent's Hospital in Linz, Austria. The sixth article from the group at the University of Texas MD Anderson Cancer Center in Houston deals with the potential and emerging utility of other PET radiotracers including amino acid derivatives, androgen receptor avid agents, hypoxia avid compounds, and other agents. In the final article, the role of PET with FDG and other tracers in radiation treatment planning and delivery in prostate cancer is discussed.

We hope that this issue of *PET Clinics* with an international list of expert contributors provides useful up-to-date information to all interested physicians, patients, and patient advocates. I take this opportunity to thank Dr. Abass Alavi for all he has contributed to the field of nuclear radiology and specifically for his invitation for me to be a Guest Editor for this issue of *PET Clinics*. I also thank Barton Dudlick for his watchful eye over the publication process from the initial concept stage to the final product. I dedicate this work to my wife, Mojgan, and my two daughters, Donya and Delara.

Hossein Jadvar, MD, PhD, MPH, MBA
University of Southern California
Keck School of Medicine
2250 Alcazar Street, CSC 102
Los Angeles, CA 90033

E-mail address:
jadvar@usc.edu (H. Jadvar)

PET Clin 4 (2009) ix
doi:10.1016/j.cpet.2009.06.004
1556-8598/09/$ – see front matter © 2009 Elsevier Inc. All rights reserved.

Role of Imaging in Prostate Cancer

Hossein Jadvar, MD, PhD, MPH, MBA[a],*,
Abass Alavi, MD, MD (Hon), Phd (Hon), DSc (Hon)[b]

KEYWORDS
- Imaging • Prostate • Cancer • MRI • Ultrasound
- CT • PET • Bone scan • Prostascint

Cancer diagnosis and therapy are undergoing rapid evolution from the current nonspecific diagnosis and treatment toward patient-specific approach to therapy. Imaging is central in this evolution because it provides accurate information on the presence and extent of disease.[1] Unprecedented developments in molecular imaging are paving the way for this new era of imaging-based cancer diagnosis and therapy. Various imaging modalities and methods may be best suited for different phases of the disease. It is best to understand the natural history of disease and its progression to tailor the imaging evaluation appropriately. In this article, we first present a brief overview of the natural history of prostate cancer before discussing the role of various imaging tools, including opportunities and challenges, for different clinical phases of this disease. In subsequent articles, we focus our attention on the role of PET in the imaging evaluation of prostate cancer.

NATURAL HISTORY OF PROSTATE CANCER

Prostate cancer is the most common cancer and the second leading cause of cancer death affecting men in the United States. In 2008, the estimated incidence of and deaths from this disease were 186,320 cases and 28,660 cases, respectively.[2] Prostate cancer is a heterogeneous disease characterized by an overall long natural history in comparison to the other solid tumors with a wide spectrum of biologic behavior that ranges between indolent and aggressive states.[3–5]

Prostate-specific antigen (PSA), a 34-kD androgen-regulated exocrine serine protease that cleaves the prostate-derived protein "seminogelin" in the seminal fluid for the liquefaction of the semen, is produced by normal and diseased prostate cells and can be measured in the serum as an "organ-specific marker" in two major isoforms of complexed to α1-antichymotrypsin and uncomplexed free PSA.[6] Various PSA parameters that have been used for monitoring include PSA density, PSA velocity, PSA half-life, PSA nadir, PSA doubling time, time to PSA elevation, age-specific PSA reference ranges, and free to total PSA ratio.[7–9] Despite the use of PSA as an "organ-specific marker," it is not ideal because of its nonspecificity and low sensitivity. PSA should not be considered a direct measure of tumor growth because the serum level is influenced by the volume of the benign epithelium, grade of carcinoma, inflammation, androgen levels, growth factors, and the extracellular matrix.[10] PSA may be undetectable or low in view of disseminated prostate cancer,[11–13] and emerging data suggest that various therapies may affect the PSA expression in a manner unrelated to the impact on tumor growth.[14–16] PSA also is frequently a source of great anxiety ("PSA-itis").[17]

In the post-PSA era, most patients (approximately 92%) present with locoregional disease,

[a] Division of Nuclear Medicine, Department of Radiology, Keck School of Medicine, University of Southern California, 2250 Alcazar Street, CSC 102, Los Angeles, CA 90033, USA
[b] Division of Nuclear Medicine, Department of Radiology, Hospital of the University of Pennsylvania, 3400 Spruce Street, 1 Donner Building, Philadelphia, PA 19104-4283, USA
* Corresponding author. Division of Nuclear Medicine, Department of Radiology, Keck School of Medicine, University of Southern California, 2250 Alcazar Street, CSC 102, Los Angeles, CA 90033, USA.
E-mail address: jadvar@usc.edu (H. Jadvar).

PET Clin 4 (2009) 135–138
doi:10.1016/j.cpet.2009.05.003

whereas metastatic disease is the initial presentation in approximately 4% of patients, with the remaining 4% of presentations classified as unknown.[1] The corresponding 5-year relative survival rates are 100% for localized/regional and 31.7% for distant disease. Despite highly successful treatments for localized prostate cancer, approximately 40% of men eventually (most within 10 years from primary treatment) experience a detectable rise in the serum PSA level (biochemical failure), which suggests that prostate cancer can metastasize relatively early in the course of the disease.[18] A portion of men with increasing serum PSA levels develop locally recurrent disease, and as many as two thirds have evidence of osseous metastatic involvement.[19–22] Patients at highest risk for bone metastases include men older than 65 years, men with high-grade, high-stage neoplasms, men who fail primary curative therapies, and men who develop PSA relapse after androgen deprivation therapy.[23–25]

Pound and colleagues[26] documented the natural history of progression to metastatic disease and death after PSA elevation after radical prostatectomy and no adjuvant hormonal therapy. A detectable serum PSA level of at least 0.2 ng/mL was considered as evidence for biochemical recurrence. The actuarial metastasis-free survival rate for all men was 82% at 15 years after surgery. The median actuarial time to metastases was 8 years from the time of PSA relapse. Once men developed metastatic disease, the median survival time to death was 5 years. The time to biochemical progression, PSA doubling time, and Gleason score were predictive of the probability and time to development of metastatic disease. The time interval from surgery to the appearance of metastatic disease was predictive of time until death. Development of hormone-refractory metastatic disease is associated with a substantially lower 1-year survival rate of only 24%.[27]

Androgens are essential for the development, growth, and maintenance of the prostate. The effects of androgens are exerted via the nuclear androgen receptor, which is a ligand-dependent (either testosterone or 5α-dihydrotestosterone) transcription activator involved in cellular proliferation and differentiation and is present in all histologic types of prostate tumors, in recurrent carcinoma, and in tumor metastases.[28–31] Almost all patients respond favorably to androgen ablation, but virtually all patients relapse to an androgen-independent clinical state. The hormone-refractory state is believed to occur via bypassing or sensitizing the androgen receptor pathway. The factors involved may be androgen receptor mutation such that the receptor is activated either promiscuously or in a ligand-independent manner. Other factors include amplification of coactivators, activation of oncogenes, and autocrine growth factor stimulation.[31]

DIAGNOSTIC IMAGING EVALUATION OF PROSTATE CANCER

Imaging evaluation of prostate cancer remains particularly challenging, which is a reflection of the clinical heterogeneity of the disease.[32–35] Initial imaging differential diagnosis may be made when suspected (eg, high serum PSA level, abnormal digital rectal examination) with ultrasound and MR imaging using endorectal probes, contrast agents, and image-guided biopsies. Imaging also provides important information on local extent of disease and examines for potential regional and distant metastatic disease in high-risk patients. The most optimal method for imaging evaluation of men with PSA relapse is unsettled, but the goal of imaging is to determine if there is recurrence in the treated prostate bed or distant disease is present (or both). Current imaging tests, including ultrasound, CT, MR imaging, bone scintigraphy, and In-111 capromab pendetide (Prostascint, Cytogen, Princeton, NJ), are not sufficiently accurate to detect local recurrence or metastatic disease in patients who have prostate cancer.[36] Such determination, however, is critical because it impacts therapeutic management, including consideration for salvage therapy for local recurrence and systemic treatment for metastatic disease.

Prostascint is a radiolabeled antibody targeted to the prostate-specific membrane antigen, which is a glycoprotein expressed in the benign and the neoplastic prostatic epithelial cells. It is up-regulated in hormone-resistant states and in metastatic disease.[37,38] Despite the relevance of prostate-specific membrane antigen in prostate cancer, Prostascint has limited predictive value in imaging the prostate fossa, particularly after radiation therapy, has low sensitivity for detecting osseous metastases, is technically demanding, and requires interpretation at sites with experience and expertise.[39,40]

Although bone scintigraphy can be useful in detecting osseous metastases, the false positive rate is high,[41] and it cannot detect soft tissue or lymph nodal involvement, which is prevalent with metastatic spread of this disease. Bone scintigraphy has limited sensitivity in detecting metastases when the serum PSA level is less than 2 ng/mL and only best correlates at high PSA levels of more than 16 ng/mL.[42,43] A "flare" phenomenon also may be observed with the initiation of hormonal ablation and even chemotherapy in the setting of clinical and serologic improvement but worsening scan pattern.[44] In patients who do not fit into this clinical scenario, however, bone scan progression may be considered when there are larger lesions, new lesions, or a combination of larger lesions and new lesions.[45] Some efforts have been made to develop methods for quantification of bone scintigraphy to facilitate quantitative determination of the extent of osseous metastatic disease and changes associated with response to treatment.[46–48] Quantitative bone scintigraphy also may have prognostic utility with the percentage of the positive area of bone metastases as an independent predictor of the disease death in patients with prostate cancer.[49,50] CT has been shown to be useful for additional evaluation of suspected skeletal metastases after bone scintigraphy by characterizing the radiographic appearance of the lesions.[51]

Newer imaging methods using lymphotropic superparamagnetic nanoparticles in conjunction with high-resolution MR imaging also may allow the detection of small and otherwise undetectable lymph node metastases in patients who have prostate cancer.[52] The exact clinical use of such diagnostic imaging approach in a diverse group of patients still needs to be determined, however.

The current availability of hybrid PET-CT imaging systems in conjunction with the most common PET radiotracer, [F-18]-fluorodeoxyglucose (FDG) have paved the way for the precise localization of metabolic abnormalities and characterization of the metabolic activity of normal and abnormal structures, thereby increasing diagnostic confidence and reducing equivocal image interpretations. Clinical use of FDG PET in oncology has included initial diagnosis, staging and restaging of cancer, detection of metastases, prediction and evaluation for therapy response, differentiation of posttherapy changes from residual or recurrent tumor, and prognostication. The clinical experience with PET and PET-CT in prostate cancer is expanding. In this issue of *PET Clinics*, we discuss the current use and emerging role of PET with FDG and other radiotracers in prostate cancer.

REFERENCES

1. Benaron DA. The future of cancer imaging. Cancer Metastasis Rev 2002;21:45–78.
2. Seer. The Surveillance, Epidemiology, and End Results Program based within the Surveillance Research Program (SRP) at the National Cancer Institute (2008). Available at: http://seer.cancer.gov/statfacts/html/prost.html. Accessed: April 6, 2009.
3. Frank IN, Graham S Jr, Nabors WL. Urologic and male genital cancers. In: Holleb AI, Fink DJ, Murphy GP, editors. Clinical oncology. Atlanta (GA): American Cancer Society; 1991. p. 280–3.
4. Kessler B, Albertsen P. The natural history of prostate cancer. Urol Clin North Am 2003;30:219–26.
5. Small EJ. Prostate cancer: incidence, management and outcomes. Drugs Aging 1998;13:71–81.
6. Lin DW, Noteboom JL, Blumenstein BA, et al. Serum percent free prostate-specific antigen in metastatic prostate cancer. Urology 1998;52:366–71.
7. Ploch NR, Brawer MK. How to use prostate-specific antigen. Urology 1994;43(2 Suppl):27–35.
8. Lukes M, Urban M, Zalesky M, et al. Prostate-specific antigen: current status. Folia Biol (Praha) 2001;47:41–9.
9. Boccon-Gibod L. [Prostate-specific antigen or PSA. Facts and probabilities]. Presse Med 1995;24:1471–2 [in French].
10. Crawford ED, DeAntoni EP, Ross CA. The role of prostate-specific antigen in the chemoprevention of prostate cancer. J Cell Biochem Suppl 1996;25:149–55.
11. Safa AA, Reese DM, Carter DM, et al. Undetectable serum prostate-specific antigen associated with metastatic prostate cancer: a case report and review of the literature. Am J Clin Oncol 1998;21:323–6.
12. Sella A, Konichezky M, Flex D, et al. Low PSA metastatic androgen-independent prostate cancer. Eur Urol 2000;38:250–4.
13. Beardo P, Fernandez PL, Corral JM, et al. Undetectable prostate specific antigen in disseminated prostate cancer. J Urol 2001 Sep;166(3):993.
14. Dreicer R. Metastatic prostate cancer: assessment of response to systemic therapy. Semin Urol Oncol 1997;15:28–32.
15. Bauer KS, Figg WD, Hamilton JM, et al. A pharmacokinetically guided phase II study of carboxy-amido-triazole in androgen-independent prostate cancer. Clin Cancer Res 1999;5(9):2324–9.
16. Horti J, Dixon SC, Logothetis C, et al. Increased transcriptional activity of PSA in the presence of TNP-470, an angiogenesis inhibitor. Br J Cancer 1999;79:1588–93.
17. Lofters A, Juffs HG, Pond GR, et al. "PSA-itis": knowledge of serum prostate specific antigen and other causes of anxiety in men with metastatic prostate cancer. J Urol 2002;168(6):2516–20.
18. Dong JT, Rinker-Schaeffer CW, Ichikawa T, et al. Prostate cancer: biology of metastasis and its clinical implications. World J Urol 1996;14:182–9.
19. Yu KK, Hawkins RA. The prostate: diagnostic evaluation of metastatic disease. Radiol Clin North Am 2000;38:139–57.
20. Carroll P. Rising PSA after a radical treatment. Eur Urol 2001;40(Suppl 2):9–16.

21. McMurtry CT, McMurtry JM. Metastatic prostate cancer: complications and treatment. J Am Geriatr Soc 2003;51:1136–42.

22. Timme TL, Satoh T, Tahir SA, et al. Therapeutic targets for metastatic prostate cancer. Curr Drug Targets 2003;4(3):251–61.

23. De la Taille A, Vancherot F, Salomon L, et al. Hormone-refractory prostate cancer: a multi-step and multi-event process. Prostate Cancer Prostatic Dis 2001;4:204–12.

24. Carlin BI, Andriole GL. The natural history, skeletal complications, and management of bone metastases in patients with prostate carcinoma. Cancer 2000;88(12 Suppl):2989–94.

25. Herold DM, Hanlon AL, Movsas B, et al. Age-related prostate cancer metastases. Urology 1998;51: 985–90.

26. Pound CR, Partin AW, Eisenberger MA, et al. Natural history of progression after PSA elevation following radical prostatectomy. JAMA 1999;281:1591–7.

27. Fossa SD, Dearnaley DP, Law M, et al. Prognostic factors in hormone-resistant progressing cancer of the prostate. Ann Oncol 1992;3:331–5.

28. Trapman J, Brinkmann AO. The androgen receptor in prostate cancer. Pathol Res Pract 1996;192:752–60.

29. Culig Z, Hobisch A, Hittmair A, et al. Androgen receptor gene mutations in prostate cancer: implications for disease progression and therapy. Drugs Aging 1997;10:50–8.

30. Culig Z, Klocker H, Bartsch G, et al. Androgen receptors in prostate cancer. Endocr Relat Cancer 2002;9:155–70.

31. Jenster G. The role of the androgen receptor in the development and progression of prostate cancer. Semin Oncol 1999;26:407–21.

32. Yu KK, Hricak H. Imaging prostate cancer. Radiol Clin North Am 2000;38:59–85.

33. Carey BM. Imaging for prostate cancer. Clin Oncol (R Coll Radiol) 2005;17:553–9.

34. Oehr P, Bouchelouche K. Imaging of prostate cancer. Curr Opin Oncol 2007;19:259–64.

35. Fuchsjager M, Shukla-Dave A, Akin O, et al. Prostate cancer imaging. Acta Radiol 2008;49:107–20.

36. Hricak H, Schoder H, Pucar D, et al. Advances in imaging in the postoperative patient with a rising prostate-specific antigen level. Semin Oncol 2003; 30:616–34.

37. Fair WR, Israeli RS, Heston WD. Prostate-specific membrane antigen. Prostate 1997;32:140–8.

38. Elgamal AA, Holmes EH, Su SL, et al. Prostate-specific membrane antigen (PSMA): current benefits and future value. Semin Surg Oncol 2000;18:10–6.

39. Haseman MK, Reed NL, Rosenthal SA. Monoclonal antibody imaging of occult prostate cancer in patients with elevated prostate-specific antigen: positron emission tomography and biopsy correlation. Clin Nucl Med 1996;21(9):704–13.

40. Haseman MK, Rosenthal SA, Polascik TJ. Capromab pendetide imaging of prostate cancer. Cancer Biother Radiopharm 2000;15(2):131–40.

41. Dotan ZA. Bone imaging in prostate cancer. Nat Clin Pract Urol 2008;5:434–44.

42. Modoni S, Calo E, Nardella G, et al. PSA and bone scintigraphy. Int J Biol Markers 1997;12:158–61.

43. Lee CT, Oesterling JE. Using prostate-specific antigen to eliminate the staging radionuclide bone scan. Urol Clin North Am 1997;24:389–94.

44. Coleman RE, Mashiter G, Whitaker KB, et al. Bone scan flare predicts successful systemic therapy for bone metastases. J Nucl Med 1988;29:1354–9.

45. Bubley GJ, Carducci M, Dahut W, et al. Eligibility and response guidelines for phase II clinical trials in androgen-independent prostate cancer: recommendations from the prostate-specific antigen working group. J Clin Oncol 1999;17:3461–7.

46. DeLuca SA, Castronovo FP, Rhea JT. The effects of chemotherapy on bony metastases as measured by quantitative skeletal imaging. Clin Nucl Med 1983;8:11–3.

47. Drelichman A, Decker DA, Al-Sarraf M, et al. Computerized bone scan: a potentially useful technique to measure response in prostate carcinoma. Cancer 1984;53:1061–5.

48. Imbriaco M, Larson SM, Yeung HW, et al. A new parameter for measuring metastatic bone involvement by prostate cancer: the bone scan index. Clin Cancer Res 1998;4:1765–72.

49. Noguchi M, Kikuchi H, Ishibashi M, et al. Percentage of the positive area of bone metastasis is an independent predictor of disease death in advanced prostate cancer. Br J Cancer 2003; 88(2):195–201.

50. Yahara J, Noghuchi M, Noda S. Quantitative evaluation of bone metastases in patients with advanced prostate cancer during systemic treatment. BJU Int 2003;92:379–84.

51. Rafii M, Firooznia H, Kramer E, et al. The role of computed tomography in evaluation of skeletal metastases. J Comput Tomogr 1988;12:19–24.

52. Harisinghani MG, Barentsz JO, Hahn PF, et al. Noninvasive detection of clinically occult lymph-node metastases in prostate cancer. N Engl J Med 2003;348(25):2491–9.

MR Imaging of the Prostate Gland

Ekta Gupta, MD, Drew A. Torigian, MD, MA*

KEYWORDS

- Prostate • Seminal tract • MR imaging
- Prostate cancer • Hematospermia

MR imaging has excellent soft tissue contrast and provides a radiation-free multiplanar anatomic evaluation of the prostate gland, seminal vesicles, ampullary portions of the vasa deferentia, and ejaculatory ducts.[1] Technical advances in MR imaging have led to the development of surface coils to improve signal-to-noise ratio and spatial resolution. The endorectal coil is a specialized surface coil that is placed in the rectum immediately adjacent to the prostate gland. This results in a small field of view leading to high spatial resolution images.[2] The standard MR imaging technique to image the prostate and seminal tract involves acquisition of multiple imaging planes through the prostate and seminal tract by means of an endorectal coil and axial images obtained with a pelvic phased-array coil through the entire pelvis.[3–5] Smooth muscle relaxant/antiperistaltic agents such as glucagon may be administered before imaging to reduce bowel motion artifact.[6,7]

The MR imaging protocol typically includes the following sequences:

Initially, sagittal localizer images are obtained to confirm optimal placement of the endorectal coil. If the endorectal coil is too low or too high, the coil position is adjusted accordingly, and localizer imaging is repeated.

Subsequently, small field-of-view axial T1-weighted images and axial, sagittal, and coronal T2-weighted images are obtained for high-resolution evaluation of the prostate and seminal tract. Fast spin echo sequences are acquired much faster than conventional spin-echo sequences, and generally are preferred, because there is less artifact from patient motion and bowel peristalsis.[3,8–10] To maximize image resolution in all three dimensions, thin slices (3 to 4 mm) and a small field of view typically are used.[11]

This is followed by large field of view images to evaluate for pelvic lymphadenopathy and osseous metastatic disease.[1,3] The use of fat suppression has not demonstrated a staging benefit compared with nonfat-suppressed T1-weighted and T2-weighted fast spin echo imaging.[2,11–13] Furthermore, lack of fat suppression allows one to improve the contrast between high signal intensity periprostatic fat and low signal intensity extracapsular tumor.[6,14]

Most studies show no superiority for contrast-enhanced MR images over T2-weighted images for evaluating the prostate.[3,11,15,16] Some utility of dynamic contrast-enhanced MRI in prostate cancer imaging has been reported in a few studies,[17–19] however, although the overall utility of dynamic contrast-enhanced MR imaging remains controversial.[20,21]

ANATOMY AND MR IMAGING APPEARANCE OF THE NORMAL PROSTATE AND SEMINAL TRACT

The prostate is an exocrine gland that surrounds the prostatic urethra at the bladder base and is located within the extraperitoneal space.[1,22,23] Approximately 70% of the prostate is composed of glandular tissue, and 30% consists of nonglandular tissue.[1,21] The normal adult prostate measures approximately 4 cm (transverse) × 3 cm (anteroposterior) × 3 cm (craniocaudad) and weighs 15

Department of Radiology, Hospital of the University of Pennsylvania, University of Pennsylvania School of Medicine, 3400 Spruce Street, Philadelphia, PA 19104, USA
* Corresponding author.
E-mail address: drew.torigian@uphs.upenn.edu (D.A. Torigian).

PET Clin 4 (2009) 139–154
doi:10.1016/j.cpet.2009.05.008

to 20 g. It functions as an accessory sex gland, and contributes approximately 0.5 mL to the normal ejaculate volume of 3.5 mL.[23]

The prostate has a base and an apex, where the prostatic base is located superiorly, and the prostatic apex is located inferiorly.[1] For anatomic division of the prostate, the zonal compartment system that has been described in the surgical and imaging literature is accepted widely.[6,21] Accordingly, the prostate is separated into the peripheral, central, and transitional zones, which constitute over 70%, 25%, and 5% of the prostate, respectively.[1,6] The peripheral zone is located posteriorly within the prostate from the base of the verumontanum to its apex; the transitional zone surrounds the proximal prostatic urethra, and the central zone surrounds the transitional zone at the prostatic base and ejaculatory ducts.[1,23,24] The central gland of the prostate is composed of the central zone and transitional zone. Seventy percent of prostate cancers arise in the peripheral zone; 20% arise in the transitional zone, and 10% arise from the central zone.[3,21] The cellular proliferation in the transition zone results in benign prostatic hyperplasia (BPH) and progressively enlarges as men age.[3,21,25]

There are two capsules in the prostate: the surgical capsule and the true capsule. The surgical capsule is a band of tissue that separates the central gland from the peripheral zone. It is a pseudocapsule and provides a cleavage plane that is used in surgical enucleation of the hyperplastic portion of the prostate.[1,23] The true (anatomic) prostatic capsule is a 2 to 3 mm fibromuscular layer that separates the peripheral zone of the prostate gland from the periprostatic soft tissues that are composed of fat and the neurovascular bundles.[1,23]

The nonglandular tissue of the prostate includes the prostatic urethra and the anterior fibromuscular stroma.[23] The anterior fibromuscular stroma forms the entire anterior surface of the prostate gland as a thick nonglandular layer of tissue and accounts for about 30% of the bulk of the prostate tissue. The prostatic ducts enter the base of the prostatic urethra and allow for the passage of prostatic secretions.[1,24]

On T1-weighted images, the normal prostate has homogenous low–intermediate signal intensity relative to skeletal muscle, with poor differentiation between the central gland and the peripheral zone. On T2-weighted images, however, the zonal anatomy of the prostate is visualized well, with diffuse homogenous high signal intensity of the peripheral zone containing thin low signal intensity linear fibrous septa, and more heterogeneous low–intermediate signal intensity of the central gland

with an intervening thin low signal intensity surgical capsule. The true capsule is low in signal intensity on T2-weighted images and separates the high signal intensity peripheral zone of the prostate from the periprostatic soft tissues. The paired neurovascular bundles contain the sympathetic nerves, arteries, and veins that supply the prostate. They are seen as low signal intensity tubular structures on T1- and T2-weighted images relative to periprostatic fat, located posterolateral to either side of the prostate gland at the 5 o'clock and 7 o'clock locations. The nerves of the neurovascular bundles typically have low signal intensity on T2-weighted images, whereas the periprostatic veins may have high signal intensity on T2-weighted images secondary to slow flow of blood.[1,3,26–28]

The prostatic urethra courses though the prostate gland from the bladder neck to the prostatic apex. The proximal periprostatic portion is located within the central prostatic gland and is usually not visible on MR imaging. Midway between the prostatic base and apex at the level of verumontanum at the junction of the central gland and peripheral zone, the prostate urethra makes an anterocaudal bend by 35° into the distal prostatic urethral portion. Through the prostate apex, the distal urethra becomes surrounded by the low signal intensity external urethral sphincter, and extends inferiorly to the penile bulb, where it is surrounded by the inferomedial aspect of the levator ani musculature.[29]

The seminal vesicles are paired accessory sex glands located superior and posterior to the prostate between the urinary bladder and the rectum in the extraperitoneal space.[1,3,22] The normal seminal vesicles average about 3.1 plus or minus 0.5 cm in length and 1.5 plus or minus 0.4 cm in width on cross-sectional imaging.[1,30] They are responsible for formation and storage of the ejaculate.

On MR imaging, the seminal vesicles have homogenous intermediate signal intensity on T1-weighted images relative to skeletal muscle, and on T2-weighted images they normally appear as convolutions of tubules that have low signal intensity walls and central high signal intensity fluid. The ampullary portions of the vasa deferentia are paired tubular structures that pass medial to the seminal vesicles, and on T2-weighted images, they have central high signal intensity fluid with thick low signal intensity walls. The caudal tip of the each seminal vesicle joins the corresponding vas deferens to form the ejaculatory duct, best seen on sagittal and coronal T2-weighted images, and which also contains high signal intensity fluid on T2-weighted images. The paired ejaculatory ducts pass through the central zone of the prostate to terminate at the verumontanum. The verumontanum generally is seen as a high signal intensity crescent in the apical portion of the prostate on T2-weighted images.[1,3,29,31] The best pulse sequence for evaluating the structures of the seminal tract is T2-weighted imaging obtained with an endorectal coil. Images in the axial plane are essential, although sagittal or coronal images are often helpful to assess the different components of the seminal tract.[1,32] **Figs. 1** and **2** show examples of the normal MR imaging appearance of the prostate and seminal tract.

NON-NEOPLASTIC DISEASES OF THE PROSTATE
Prostatitis

Epidemiologic studies have confirmed that prostatitis is common, with a prevalence of 2% to 16%.[33–35] Although prostatitis can occur at any age, its incidence increases with age.[33] The National Institutes of Health classification of prostatitis has been accepted internationally and includes four categories.[36,37] Briefly, they include:

Category 1, acute bacterial prostatitis that is characterized by acute bacterial urinary tract infection and presents with constitutional symptoms, positive cultures of urine or prostatic secretions, and inflammatory cells in prostatic secretions.

Category 2, chronic bacterial prostatitis that has a more insidious onset and presents with relapsing or persistent urinary tract infections and irritative or obstructive genitourinary symptoms.

Category 3, chronic prostatitis/chronic pelvic pain syndrome that is characterized by chronic pelvic pain symptoms in the absence of urinary tract infection, with or without inflammation. The inflammatory type presents with genitourinary or rectal pain or voiding symptoms, and the prostatic fluid contains inflammatory cells, whereas in the noninflammatory type, the prostatic fluid has no leukocytes, and the presenting symptoms are similar, although pelvic pain is usually the predominant complaint.

Category 4, asymptomatic inflammatory prostatitis that accounts for men who have prostatic inflammation detected during the evaluation of another disorder.

Of the men presenting with symptoms of prostatitis, most have nonbacterial prostatitis or chronic pelvic pain syndrome, whereas only 5% to 10% have acute or chronic bacterial prostatitis.[36]

Imaging rarely is performed in the evaluation of affected men.[3] For example, in patients who have symptoms of chronic prostatitis that are resistant to therapy, MR imaging may be

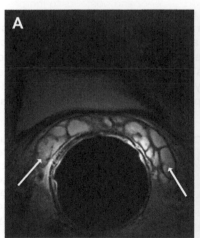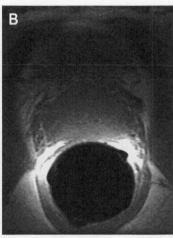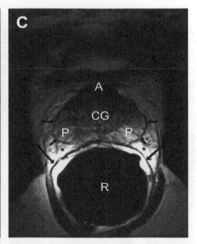

Fig. 1. Normal MR imaging anatomy of prostate and seminal tract. (*A*) Axial T2 weighted endorectal MR image shows seminal vesicles (*arrows*) with low signal intensity walls and central high signal intensity fluid. (*B*) Axial T1 weighted endorectal MR image shows homogeneous low–intermediate signal intensity of prostate relative to skeletal muscle. (*C*) Axial T2 weighted endorectal MR image shows homogeneous high signal intensity of peripheral zone (P) containing thin low signal intensity linear fibrous septa and more heterogeneous low–intermediate signal intensity central gland (CG). Also note thick low signal intensity anterior fibromuscular stroma (*A*), true prostatic capsule (*short arrows*) with low signal intensity, rectoprostatic angles (*), low signal intensity perirectal fascia (*long arrows*), and very low signal intensity void in rectum (R) in location of endorectal coil placement.

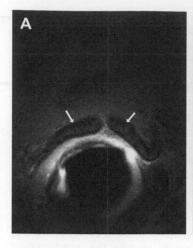
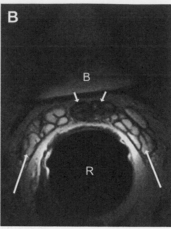

Fig. 2. Normal MR imaging anatomy of seminal tract. (*A, B*) Axial T2 weighted endorectal MR images demonstrate thick-walled ampullary portions of vasa deferentia (*short arrows*) located medial to seminal vesicles (*long arrows*). Note high signal intensity fluid in bladder (*B*) and very low signal intensity in rectum (R) caused by endorectal coil placement.

performed to exclude an abscess or associated structural abnormality.[3,38] Detection of prostatitis on MR imaging remains a challenge.[33] On MR imaging, the size and signal intensity of the prostate gland may be normal.[39] One, however, alternatively may see low T1- and T2-weighted signal intensity in the peripheral zone, which may be focal or diffuse (**Fig. 3**), usually without contour deformation of the prostate. A nodular appearance mimicking prostate carcinoma also may occur, however.[1,40] MR spectroscopic imaging of regions of chronic prostatitis can demonstrate metabolic abnormalities (such as elevated choline levels and reduced citrate levels) that mimic those of prostate cancer.[33,40]

Prostatic and Seminal Tract Cystic Lesions

Cystic lesions of the prostate and seminal tract can be divided into congenital and acquired lesions. Congenital cystic lesions include utricular, Müllerian duct, ejaculatory duct, and seminal vesicle cysts. Acquired cystic lesions include retention cysts, cystic BPH, ejaculatory duct cysts, cystic carcinoma, and prostatic abscess.[41]

MR imaging can be very helpful in demonstrating the exact anatomic location and extent of a cystic lesion with respect to the prostate gland and seminal tract.[42,43] Simple fluid within cystic lesions has low signal intensity on T1-weighted images and high signal intensity on T2-weighted images, whereas proteinaceous or hemorrhagic fluid may demonstrate variably increased signal intensity on T1-weighted images and variably decreased signal intensity on T2-weighted images.[1]

Congenital cysts

Midline cysts The two major types of midline prostatic cysts are the utricular and müllerian duct cysts. These occur in the prostate gland in 1% to 5% of adults and may cause irritative or obstructive lower urinary tract symptoms caused by compression of the prostatic urethra or ejaculatory ducts,

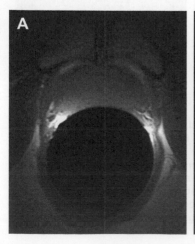
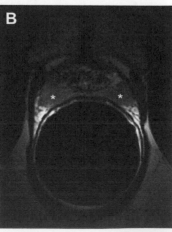

Fig. 3. Chronic prostatitis. (*A*) Axial T1 weighted endorectal MR image reveals homogeneous low–intermediate signal intensity of prostate similar to skeletal muscle. (*B*) Axial T2 weighted endorectal MR image reveals diffuse low signal intensity throughout peripheral zone (*) caused by chronic prostatitis.

male infertility if there is ejaculatory duct or vas deferens obstruction, or other symptoms and signs such as pain, fever, hematuria, or hematospermia if infected or hemorrhagic. At digital rectal examination, a cystic rectal lesion may be palpated.[1]

The utricular cyst arises from the utricle (derived from the urogenital sinus), is endodermal in origin, may contain spermatozoa at aspiration, and may communicate with the ejaculatory duct or posterior urethra. As opposed to an enlarged utricle, which is common in childhood and may be associated with intersex problems, cryptorchidism, hypospadias, or other conditions, the utricular cyst often is detected incidentally at imaging in adults and is not associated with other congenital conditions. Utricular cysts are small, usually 8 to 10 mm long, and pear-shaped, and they have no extension above the base of the prostate.[1,3,40]

The müllerian duct cyst is a congenital cystic remnant formed from the caudal ends of fused Müllerian ducts, is mesodermal in origin, and is the homolog of the paranephric duct remnants and uterus. It generally is not associated with intersex problems, hypospadias, or other abnormalities. It generally presents later in life than utricular cysts, and does not contain spermatozoa or fructose at aspiration, as it does not communicate with the urethra, ejaculatory duct, or seminal vesicles.[1] Diagnosis often is made by detection of a calcified calculus in the retrovesical cavity that does not communicate with the bladder.[41,42] Calculi may lead to hemorrhage into the cyst, which can be seen as high signal intensity on T1-weighted images.[41] Müllerian cysts tend to be larger, have a teardrop shape, and may extend beyond the posterosuperior margin of the prostate (**Fig. 4**).[3]

On MR imaging, utricular and Müllerian duct cysts typically occur in the midline of the prostate.[44,45] Sometimes, sagittal images might be useful to demonstrate a possible connection between the cyst and the posterior urethra, as it would be expected for a utricular cyst.[42] Lateral bowing of the ejaculatory ducts or identification of the ejaculatory ducts within the cyst walls may be seen in association with utricular and Müllerian duct cysts, and may be useful to separate these from ejaculatory duct cysts.[1]

Paramedian cysts Ejaculatory duct cysts are located laterally but close to the midline; they contain spermatozoa at aspiration and are rare.[1,41] They are usually the result of partial distal obstruction of the ejaculatory duct that may be congenital or acquired secondary to inflammation.[1,44] These cysts when small usually are not associated with symptoms, although large cysts can be associated with hematospermia, ejaculatory pain, perineal pain, and dysuria.[44,46] On MR imaging, ejaculatory duct cysts usually appear as round or oval thin-walled unilocular cystic lesions, typically in a paramedian location along the expected course of the ejaculatory ducts, and they may contain low signal intensity calculi. They typically contain fluid with low signal intensity on T1-weighted images and high signal intensity on T2-weighted images.[1,41,44,47]

Lateral cysts Seminal vesicle cysts usually present in the third decade of life, are an uncommon congenital abnormality, and frequently are

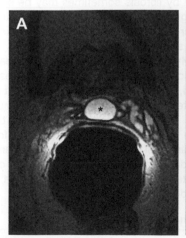 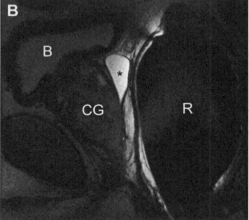

Fig. 4. Müllerian duct cyst. (*A, B*) Axial (*A*) and sagittal (*B*) T2 weighted endorectal MR images show well-circumscribed thin-walled teardrop-shaped lesion within midline of prostate containing high signal intensity fluid (*) caused by Müllerian duct cyst. Note enlargement of central gland (CG) caused by benign prostatic hyperplasia. *Abbreviations:* B, bladder; R, rectum.

associated with autosomal dominant polycystic kidney disease, ipsilateral renal anomalies such as renal agenesis, ipsilateral congenital absence of the vas deferens, or ectopic ureteral insertion into mesonephric duct derivatives such as the seminal vesicle or ejaculatory duct.[48–51] Sometimes they may be acquired from prior infection or inflammation, and clinically they may present with symptoms of urinary tract obstruction, epididymitis, prostatitis, or painful ejaculation. The cyst fluid contains fructose and spermatozoa at aspiration, as they communicate with the seminal tract.[1,32] On MR imaging, they appear as thin-walled unilocular cystic lesions within the seminal vesicle posterolateral to the urinary bladder, and they may be associated with ipsilateral ejaculatory duct dilation or may protrude into the urinary bladder, mimicking the appearance of an ectopic ureterocele. A distal dilated ectopic ureter also may be seen when present, and this sometimes may drain into the seminal vesicle cyst. Also, an abnormality of the ipsilateral kidney may be visualized on large field-of-view localizer images.[1,49,51]

Acquired cystic lesions

Retention cysts These acquired cysts result from obstruction of prostatic glandular ductules causing dilation of the glandular acini, usually occur in the fifth and sixth decades of life, and rarely are these symptomatic. They can occur in any zone of the prostate; they are usually round, smooth-walled, and unilocular, and they do not contain spermatozoa.[41,44,45]

Cystic degeneration of benign prostatic hyperplasia BPH is very common, and cystic changes are common within the hyperplastic nodules of BPH. As such, this is the most common cystic lesion of the prostate, and it is located in the transitional zone. Although BPH often results in obstructive symptoms, the cystic foci themselves are usually small and rarely cause symptoms.[41,44]

Cystic or necrotic prostate carcinoma Prostate carcinoma presenting as a cystic lesion rather than a solid lesion is rare. It should be suspected, however, when there is a rapid growth in size of a cystic lesion in the prostate, or presence of a solid component, cyst wall irregularity, or cyst wall nodularity.[41,52]

Prostatic abscess Prostatic abscesses are uncommon cystic lesions, and they usually result from inadequately treated acute bacterial prostatitis. They usually are seen in the fifth and sixth decades of life, mainly affecting diabetic and immunosuppressed patients. *Escherichia coli* is the most frequent causative organism.[44,53] On digital rectal examination, clinical detection is possible when a soft prostate is palpated with a fluctuating collection, although this is an uncommon finding. The differentiation between prostatitis and an abscess is usually difficult on a clinical basis, as the symptoms and signs are frequently similar.[53,54] Early diagnosis is important, however, because the treatment of prostatic abscess usually consists of drainage and antibiotic therapy.[53–55] Although not much has been reported about the MR imaging appearance of the prostate abscess, it generally has variable signal intensity fluid on T1- and T2-weighted images depending on the proteinaceous and cellular content, with multiple internal septations and a thick enhancing rim, sometimes with very low signal intensity foci of gas also noted.[53,56]

OTHER INFECTIOUS DISEASES OF THE PROSTATE

Schistosomal (bilharzial) infection of the prostate and seminal vesicles is seldom found in clinical practice, but it has been reported to be present in up to 58% of men living in endemic areas at autopsy.[57,58] It is secondary to parasitic infection by trematodes of the *Schistosoma* genus, most commonly *S haematobium*, and it should be considered when calcifications of the prostate gland, seminal vesicles, or bladder wall are seen at transrectal ultrasonography (TRUS) or CT, or when a change in quality of the ejaculate to a yellow color or watery consistency is the chief complaint, particularly in young men with a recent history of travel to endemic areas.[57–61] Calcifications frequently are not seen well on MR imaging, although occasional dilation of the ejaculatory ducts or seminal vesicles caused y distal obstruction by fibrosis sometimes may be seen.[58,59] The diagnosis can be established definitively through microscopic visualization of *Schistosoma* eggs in the seminal fluid.[58,59,62]

Mycobacterial infection also can lead to calcification of the prostate, seminal vesicles, or bladder wall, best seen at TRUS or CT, and it may be detected in conjunction with streaky low signal intensity on T2-weighted images within the prostate (the watermelon skin sign), abscess formation, or findings of urinary tract involvement including bladder wall or ureteral thickening or calcification, ureteral stricture formation, and a decreased bladder capacity.[63–68]

Amyloidosis

Amyloidosis, an idiopathic disease, is characterized by extracellular deposition of abnormal proteinaceous material, and it may be systemic or localized. Systemic forms usually are subdivided based on the type of rigid nonbranching fibrils that are deposited. The primary or idiopathic form of amyloidosis that is associated with multiple myeloma involves deposition of monoclonal antibody light (AL) chain, whereas the secondary form of amyloidosis that is associated with chronic inflammation involves deposition of amyloid A protein (AA). Localized amyloidosis mainly affects the brain, heart, or pancreas, with only rare involvement of the lower urinary tract and prostate occurring.[69,70] In a study by Wilson and colleagues,[71] amyloid deposits were detected in 10% of prostatic material submitted from a random population and in 47% from a selected population with multiple myeloma and primary amyloidosis. Some studies suggest that amyloidosis of the prostate may increase serum prostate-specific antigen (PSA) levels because of an associated inflammatory response, although this in part may be caused by coexistent BPH.

On MR imaging, amyloidosis often mimics the appearance of prostate cancer. Diagnosis is made through prostatic biopsy when positive staining with Congo red under microscopy with typical green birefringence in polarized light is observed.[1] Usually, localized prostatic involvement alone does not require treatment, although systemic amyloidosis involving multiple organs may warrant therapy. In the setting of an elevated serum PSA, clinicians first must exclude the presence of prostate cancer even in the setting of known amyloidosis.[69]

Seminal vesicle amyloidosis is a more common finding than prostatic amyloidosis, particularly in the elderly, and it rarely presents clinically. In localized or senile seminal vesicle amyloidosis, localized amyloid deposits occur subepithelially in the lamina propria of the seminal vesicles, usually in distinct foci, whereas in systemic amyloidosis of the seminal vesicles, amyloid deposits also may occur in the walls of the vessels or in the muscular tissue. On MR imaging, nodular thickening of the convolutions of the seminal vesicles or focal or diffuse decreased signal intensity on T2-weighted images may be seen, potentially mimicking the spread of prostate carcinoma to the seminal vesicles. Sometimes, associated high T1-weighted signal intensity seminal vesicle hemorrhage may be detected also. Hematospermia caused by localized amyloid deposition in the seminal vesicles is intermittent and does not require therapeutic intervention other than patient reassurance and long-term follow-up.[1]

Calculi

Calculi, when visualized, typically appear as very low signal intensity foci on T1- and T2-weighted images within the prostate gland or seminal tract.[1] More than 50% of prostatic calculi are composed in part by components of urine, suggesting a reflux phenomenon. As such, seminal vesicle calculi also may be caused in part by a similar reflux phenomenon or may be caused by stasis with concretion of complex fluid and debris.[46,72]

Hematospermia

Hematospermia (HS) is an anxiety-provoking but generally benign and self-limited condition that is associated with significant underlying pathology infrequently. Although it is not uncommon, the exact prevalence and incidence of HS are unknown.[73] Most men who have HS are young (younger than 40 years), and HS may occur either as a single episode or repeatedly over time.[73–75] It may arise in association with pathology involving the prostate, seminal tract, urinary bladder, urethra, epididymides, or testes.[22] The most common entities in men who have HS include prior prostatic biopsy, prostatic calculi, BPH, and inflammation/infection such as chronic prostatitis or seminal vesiculitis, although most cases are idiopathic, with the most likely site of origin occurring in the seminal vesicles.[1] Most men who have HS can be managed conservatively, as there is a low risk of serious underlying pathology.[74] In a study by Han and colleagues involving 26,126 men who underwent routine prostate cancer screening, however, only 0.5% had HS, but 14% of patients who had HS were diagnosed with prostate cancer. Therefore, when a man 40 years old or older presents with HS, screening for prostate carcinoma may be prudent.[76]

Through endorectal coil MR imaging, Lencioni and colleagues[77] showed abnormalities in 54% of 90 men who had HS, including dilation of the seminal vesicles or ejaculatory duct in 34%, hemorrhage within these structures in 25%, utricular cysts in 9%, ejaculatory duct cysts in 7%, and seminal vesicle calculi in 8%. Maeda and colleagues[39] showed abnormalities in 94% of 15 men who had HS, including seminal vesicle cysts or dilation in 87%, unilateral subacute hemorrhage in 73%, and midline prostatic cysts in 20%. Hemorrhage within the prostate and seminal tract tends to be visualized in its subacute form in men who had HS, and on MR imaging typically has high signal intensity on T1-weighted images and variable T2-weighted signal intensity (**Figs. 5** and **6**).[1,78] Endorectal MR imaging may play an important role in the diagnostic workup of men who have HS, particularly in those who are at least 40 years old, have other associated symptoms or signs of disease, or have persistent HS. Specific therapeutic

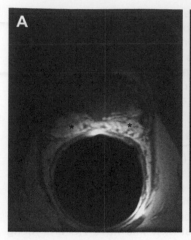
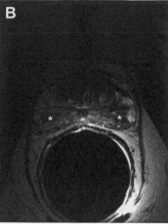

Fig. 5. Prostatic hemorrhage. (*A*) Axial T1 weighted endorectal MR image demonstrates areas of high signal intensity within peripheral zone (*) caused by subacute hemorrhage. (*B*) Axial T2 weighted endorectal MR image demonstrates corresponding low signal intensity (*) of these areas relative to normal peripheral zone.

interventions may be used if certain treatable underlying pathologies are detected. Otherwise, management with routine clinical evaluation, watchful waiting, and reassurance generally suffices.[1]

Benign Prostatic Hypertrophy

BPH affects more than 70% of men over age 60 and as many of 90% of men over age 70. Although the exact etiology of BPH is unknown, it probably is associated with hormonal changes that occur with aging. It originates within the transitional zone of the prostate, and consists of nodular hypertrophy of the fibrous, muscular, and glandular tissue elements, with resultant enlargement of the central gland.[1,33]

On MR imaging, heterogenous nodular enlargement of the central gland caused by hypointense stromal-dominant foci and hyperintense glandular-rich nodular foci on T2-weighted images, sometimes with compression of the peripheral zone or mass effect on the bladder base, may be visualized. In addition, an overall increase in prostatic size and volume often is seen, sometimes with bulges in the prostatic capsule without disruption caused by nodular foci of BPH (see **Fig. 6**). Associated diverticulum formation, trabeculation, or diffuse wall thickening of the urinary bladder may be visualized also because of chronic outlet obstruction.[1]

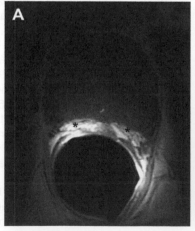
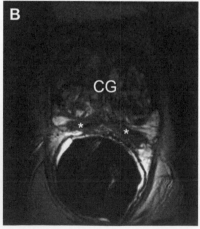

Fig. 6. Prostatic hemorrhage and benign prostatic hyperplasia (BPH). (*A*) Axial T1 weighted endorectal MR image reveals areas of high signal intensity within peripheral zone (*) caused by subacute hemorrhage. Note marked enlargement of overall prostate size. (*B*) Axial T2 weighted endorectal MR image reveals low signal intensity (*) of areas of hemorrhage relative to normal peripheral zone. Also note heterogeneous nodular enlargement of central gland (CG) caused by BPH.

Neoplastic Disease of the Prostate

Prostate adenocarcinoma

Prostate adenocarcinoma accounts for 95% of all prostate malignancies, and it is the most commonly diagnosed malignancy and the second leading cause of cancer death in American men.[79,80] In 2008, prostate cancer was diagnosed in over 186,000 men in the United States, and accounted for more than 28,000 deaths annually.[81,82] Prostate cancer is rare under the age of 40, and its incidence increases exponentially with age.[83] African American men have an increased incidence of prostate cancer and almost twice the mortality compared with Caucasian men.[84] An estimated 95% of cases of prostate cancer are expected to be diagnosed at local or regional stages, for which the 5-year relative survival approaches 100%.[81]

The diagnosis of prostate cancer is based mainly on a combination of digital rectal examination, measurement of serum PSA levels, and biopsy guided by TRUS.[85] Once the diagnosis of prostate cancer is made, the primary goal of local staging is to assist in treatment planning by differentiating patients with organ confined disease (stage T1 to T2), who can be treated with surgery or radiation therapy, from those with extracapsular extension of tumor or seminal vesicle invasion (stage T3) or malignant lymphadenopathy or bone marrow metastases (stage T4) who are not surgical candidates but who can be treated with radiation therapy, hormonal therapy, or both.[3,11,85] Most (70%) prostate cancers originate from the peripheral zone, but up to 30% occur within the transitional zone.[21,86,87]

On MR imaging, prostate adenocarcinoma is typically intermediate in signal intensity on T1-weighted images and low in signal intensity on T2-weighted images relative to the normal peripheral zone (**Fig. 7**).[83,88–90] Low signal intensity within the peripheral zone on T2-weighted images, however, also can be seen in other non-neoplastic etiologies such as prostatitis, postbiopsy hemorrhage, postradiation fibrosis, and following hormonal therapy.[6,21,91] Postbiopsy hemorrhage can be differentiated from tumor by accompanying high signal intensity on T1-weighted images.[21] Despite the nonspecificity of MR imaging, endorectal MR imaging combined with large field-of-view pelvic MR imaging with a body surface coil sorts patients into two groups: those who are potential surgical candidates and those who are not.[6,91]

Obliteration of the rectoprostatic angle, asymmetry of the neurovascular bundles, and direct invasion of adjacent organs (eg, the seminal vesicles or urinary bladder) by low signal intensity soft tissue on T1-weighted and T2-weighted images are specific findings of extracapsular spread of tumor (**Fig. 8**).[1,92,93] Pelvic lymphadenopathy (**Fig. 9**) and osseous metastases (**Fig. 10**) also may be seen when there is metastatic disease.[1] MR imaging has been reported to have a range of sensitivities (13% to 95%) and specificities (49% to 97%) for extracapsular tumor extension detection, and a similar range of sensitivities (23% to 80%) and specificities (81% to 99%) for detecting seminal vesicle invasion by tumor.[20,94] The overall accuracy of MR imaging in the staging of prostate cancer is 54% to 93%,[20,95–100] with sensitivity of 51% to 89% and specificity of 67% to 87%.[101]

Evaluation of transitional zone prostate cancer with MR imaging is more difficult, as the central gland (often with BPH) has a greater percentage of fibrous stroma than the peripheral zone, which results in heterogeneous and lower T2-weighted

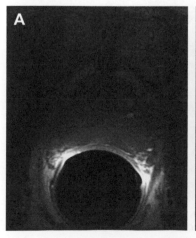
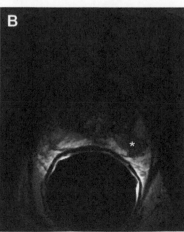

Fig. 7. Peripheral zone prostate carcinoma without extracapsular extension. (*A*) Axial T1 weighted endorectal MR image shows homogeneous low–intermediate signal intensity of prostate similar to skeletal muscle. (*B*) Axial T2 weighted endorectal MR image shows focal low signal intensity (*) within left posterolateral peripheral zone of prostatic midgland caused by prostate carcinoma. Note lack of extension of soft tissue through true prostatic capsule into the adjacent rectoprostatic angle.

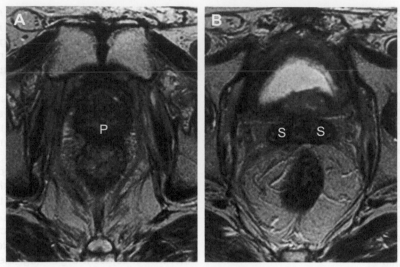

Fig. 8. Peripheral zone prostate carcinoma with seminal vesicle invasion. (A, B) Axial T2 weighted pelvic MR images show low signal intensity in enlarged prostate (P) and in enlarged seminal vesicles (S) with loss of normal convolutions and high signal intensity fluid, in keeping with extracapsular spread of prostate carcinoma.

signal intensity.[6,94,102] Certain MR imaging findings, however, may suggest the diagnosis of transitional zone cancer, including:

An area of homogenous low T2-weighted signal intensity in the central gland

Ill-defined margins

Lack of a low signal intensity rim (because BPH nodules typically have well-defined margins with a visible capsule)

Alenticular shape (because BPH nodules are typically round)

Urethral or anterior fibromuscular stromal invasion

Interruption of the surgical capsule **(Fig. 11)**[20,102]

Akin and colleagues[102] reported that prostate volume was an important factor for detecting transitional zone cancers, such that the accuracy of cancer detection increased when the tumor volume was at least 0.77 cm^3.

Technical advances in MR imaging over the last 20 years have led to development of newer

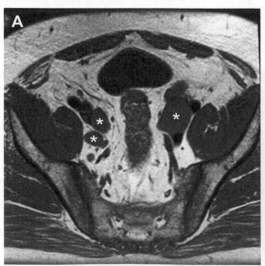
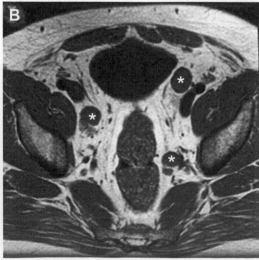

Fig. 9. Metastatic pelvic lymphadenopathy caused by prostate carcinoma. (A, B) Axial T1 weighted pelvic MR images reveal bilateral enlarged internal and external iliac chain lymph nodes (*) caused by metastatic disease.

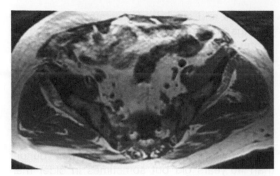

Fig. 10. Bone marrow metastatic disease caused by prostate carcinoma. Axial T1 weighted pelvic MR image shows multiple low signal intensity lesions throughout iliac bones and sacrum caused by sclerotic bone marrow metastases.

functional imaging modalities to assess tumor in the prostate. These functional MR imaging techniques include in vivo MR spectroscopy, diffusion weighted imaging (DWI), and dynamic contrast-enhanced (DCE) perfusion MR imaging.

MR spectroscopy provides information on prostate metabolism by displaying the amounts and relative ratios of citrate, choline, and creatine levels in the prostate. Normal prostatic tissue has high levels of citrate, whereas reduced levels of citrate and increased levels of choline are indicative of prostate cancer. Because choline and creatine peaks at 1.5T MR spectroscopy may overlap,

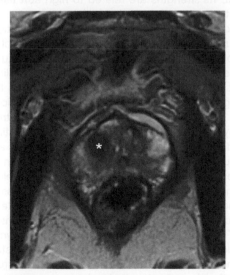

Fig. 11. Central gland prostate carcinoma without extracapsular extension. Axial T2 weighted pelvic MR image demonstrates focal homogeneous low signal intensity within right central gland of prostate (*) with ill-defined margins and lack of low signal intensity rim caused by prostate carcinoma.

a commonly used marker for cancer is the ratio of the sum of choline and creatine levels to citrate levels.[21,94,103–105] Some studies report that addition of MR spectroscopy to MR imaging improves cancer volume measurement and localization within the prostate, cancer aggressiveness, and extracapsular tumor extension.[8,106–113] Recent retrospective studies in patients who had prostate cancer confirmed at surgical pathology found that combined MR imaging/MR spectroscopy had sensitivity of 42% to 83%, specificity of 81% to 89%, accuracy of 74% to 85%, positive predictive value (PPV) of 81% to 93%, and negative predictive value (NPV) of 50% to 86% in staging prostate cancer.[103] A recent prospective multicenter study reported by Weinreb and colleagues,[114] however, showed that the accuracy of combined 1.5 T endorectal coil MR imaging/MR spectroscopy for sextant localization of peripheral zone prostate cancer is equal to that of MR imaging alone.

Introduction of ultrafast echo planar sequences in prostate MR imaging has led to the introduction of DWI, which provides contrast through measurement of the diffusion properties of water molecules within tissues.[33,94] In general, cancer tends to have more restricted diffusion of water molecules than does normal tissue because of excesses of intracellular and intercellular membranes and higher cell densities.[21,94] This leads to a decrease in signal intensity on apparent diffusion coefficient (ADC) map images and DWI.[21,103] So far, very few studies describe the use of this technique in prostate cancer. For example, Morgan and colleagues in a prospective study of 56 patients showed that for an experienced reader in prostate cancer detection, there was an improvement in sensitivity for the detection of prostate cancer (73.2% for combined MR imaging/DWI compared with 50% for MR imaging alone). The specificity, accuracy, PPV, and NPV also improved from 79.6% to 80.8%, 66.6% to 77.5%, 65.7% to 74.8%, and 67.1% to 79.5%, respectively.[115]

DCE perfusion MR imaging takes advantage of the presence of angiogenesis as a diagnostic marker for cancer, and it is performed by obtaining multiple T1-weighted images through one or more slices of the prostate over time following the intravenous administration of gadolinium-based contrast material.[20,105,116] Engelbrecht and colleagues[17] reported that the relative peak enhancement was the most accurate perfusion parameter for detecting cancer in the peripheral zone and central gland, with areas under the receiver operating characteristic (ROC) curves of 0.93 and 0.82, respectively. Kim and colleagues[18] reported that wash-in rate of contrast was more accurate than T2-weighted imaging alone for the detecting prostate cancer in the peripheral zone, although they noted overlap between the perfusional properties of normal tissue and cancer. Futterer and colleagues, in a prospective study of 34 patients, showed that for localization of tumor volumes of greater than or equal to 0.5 cm^3, addition of T1-weighted DCE MR imaging to T2-weighted imaging led to an increase in sensitivity from 69% to 95%, and increases in specificity (80% to 96%) and accuracy (81% to 93%). For assessing the extracapsular extension of tumor, the sensitivity, specificity, accuracy, PPV, and NPV of combined MR imaging and DCE MR imaging were 82% to 91%, 95%, 95% to 96%, 90% to 91%, and 91% to 95%, respectively.[117] Overall, there remains debate regarding the best image acquisition and postprocessing protocols and the optimal perfusion parameter to distinguish cancer from normal tissue.[21,94]

Another goal of MR imaging in the setting of prostate cancer is to improve the detection of pelvic lymph node metastases through the use of lymph node-specific superparamagnetic iron oxide particles as negative contrast agents.[2,20] This goal is an important one, as lymph node involvement by tumor changes the tumor stage, treatment options, and patient prognosis.[2] Currently available treatment protocols for prostate cancer patients exclude a surgical cure if there are even micrometastases in a single lymph node.[118,119] Also, routine MR imaging relies mainly on lymph node size (a short-axis diameter of greater than or equal to 10 mm) to determine whether a lymph node is pathologic in nature, but it is limited in sensitivity and specificity for detecting metastatic disease.[2,116,118]

After superparamagnetic iron oxide particles are administered intravenously, they are taken up by macrophages in normal-functioning lymph nodes, leading to a loss of signal intensity on T2-weighted fast spin echo and T2*-weighted gradient echo images. Foci of metastatic disease within lymph nodes, where normal macrophages are replaced, will not take up the particles, however, and thus will not decrease in signal intensity.[2,18,20,120] Harisinghani and colleagues reported the use of lymphotropic superparamagnetic iron particle MR imaging to identify prostate cancer metastasis to lymph nodes; 71.4% of nodes with histopathologically detected metastases were of normal size. The sensitivity and specificity for the detection of metastasis were 35.4% and 90.4%, respectively, for conventional MR imaging, and 99.5% and 97.8%, respectively, for lymphotropic superparamagnetic iron particle MR imaging.[120]

Although a few studies suggest that functional MR imaging techniques may improve the diagnosis and staging of prostate cancer, these findings require confirmation by larger-scale multicenter randomized studies to compare these techniques. As of yet, there are no guidelines with regard to which functional MR imaging techniques are best for a specific clinical situation.[21,103]

Prostate sarcoma

Sarcoma of the prostate is rare. The two most common subtypes are leiomyosarcoma and rhabdomyosarcoma.[3] It usually occurs in men younger than 40 years old but sometimes in older men (especially those who have prostate leiomyosarcoma). Clinical symptoms may include urinary retention, hematuria, hematospermia, rectal pain, or a palpable rectal or abdominal mass.

On MR imaging, it often presents as a large bulky heterogenous tumor mass with variable signal intensity on T1- and T2-weighted images secondary to variable amounts of necrosis and cystic change with diffuse infiltration of the prostate gland and periprostatic tissues. It often is characterized by rapid and extensive local and distant spread of disease also.[121–125] Negative margins at the time of surgery and absence of metastatic disease at presentation are the two most important factors that predict long-term survival.[126]

SUMMARY

MR imaging is a powerful imaging modality for comprehensive structural evaluation of anatomy and pathology of the prostate gland and seminal tract. Its strengths are related to high soft tissue contrast resolution, high spatial resolution, and a lack of ionizing radiation, whereas its limitations are related mainly to insensitivity for the detection of pathology at the molecular level and frequent nonspecificity of structural imaging abnormalities that are encountered. Technical advances in MR imaging have led to development of functional MR imaging techniques such as MR spectroscopy, DWI, and DCE perfusion imaging, potentially leading to increased sensitivity, specificity, and accuracy of detection and characterization of disease processes. With potential future development and implementation of positron emission tomography (PET)/MR imaging hybrid systems for clinical or research purposes, the strengths of PET and MR imaging can be combined in a synergistic fashion to optimally evaluate the prostate gland and seminal tract at the structural, gross functional, and molecular levels.

REFERENCES

1. Turigian DA, Ramchandani P. Hematospermia: imaging findings. Abdom Imaging 2007;32(1):29–49.

2. Heenan SD. Magnetic resonance imaging in prostate cancer. Prostate Cancer Prostatic Dis 2004; 7(4):282–8.

3. Siegelman ES. Body MRI. Philadelphia: Elsevier Inc.; 2005.

4. Hricak H, White S, Vigneron D, et al. Carcinoma of the prostate gland: MR imaging with pelvic phased-array coils versus integrated endorectal–pelvic phased-array coils. Radiology 1994;193(3): 703–9.

5. Schnall MD, Lenkinski RE, Pollack HM, et al. Prostate: MR imaging with an endorectal surface coil. Radiology 1989;172(2):570–4.

6. Siegelman ES. Magnetic resonance imaging of the prostate. Semin Roentgenol 1999;34(4):295–312.

7. Chernish SM, Maglinte DD. Glucagon: common untoward reactions—review and recommendations. Radiology 1990;177(1):145–6.

8. Kurhanewicz J, Vigneron DB, Males RG, et al. The prostate: MR imaging and spectroscopy. Present and future. Radiol Clin North Am 2000;38(1): 115–38.

9. Nghiem HV, Herfkens RJ, Francis IR, et al. The pelvis: T2-weighted fast spin echo MR imaging. Radiology 1992;185(1):213–7.

10. Constable RT, Smith RC, Gore JC. Signal-to-noise and contrast in fast spin echo (FSE) and inversion recovery FSE imaging. J Comput Assist Tomogr 1992;16(1):41–7.

11. Yu KK, Hricak H. Imaging prostate cancer. Radiol Clin North Am 2000;38(1):59–85.

12. Tsuda K, Yu KK, Coakley FV, et al. Detection of extracapsular extension of prostate cancer: role of fat suppression endorectal MRI. J Comput Assist Tomogr 1999;23(1):74–8.

13. Mirowitz SA, Heiken JP, Brown JJ. Evaluation of fat saturation technique for T2-weighted endorectal coil MRI of the prostate. Magn Reson Imaging 1994;12(5):743–7.

14. Ikonen S, Karkkainen P, Kivisaari L, et al. Magnetic resonance imaging of clinically localized prostatic cancer. J Urol 1998;159(3):915–9.

15. Huch Boni RA, Boner JA, Lutolf UM, et al. Contrast-enhanced endorectal coil MRI in local staging of prostate carcinoma. J Comput Assist Tomogr 1995;19(2):232–7.

16. Mirowitz SA, Brown JJ, Heiken JP. Evaluation of the prostate and prostatic carcinoma with gadolinium-enhanced endorectal coil MR imaging. Radiology 1993;186(1):153–7.

17. Engelbrecht MR, Huisman HJ, Laheij RJ, et al. Discrimination of prostate cancer from normal peripheral zone and central gland tissue by using dynamic contrast-enhanced MR imaging. Radiology 2003;229(1):248–54.

18. Kim JK, Hong SS, Choi YJ, et al. Wash-in rate on the basis of dynamic contrast-enhanced MRI: usefulness for prostate cancer detection and localization. J Magn Reson Imaging 2005;22(5): 639–46.

19. Jackson AS, Reinsberg SA, Sohaib SA, et al. Dynamic contrast-enhanced MRI for prostate cancer localization. Br J Radiol 2009;82(974):148–56.

20. Hricak H, Choyke PL, Eberhardt SC, et al. Imaging prostate cancer: a multidisciplinary perspective. Radiology 2007;243(1):28–53.

21. Choi YJ, Kim JK, Kim N, et al. Functional MR imaging of prostate cancer. Radiographics 2007; 27(1):63–75 [discussion: 7].

22. Munkelwitz R, Krasnokutsky S, Lie J, et al. Current perspectives on hematospermia: a review. J Androl 1997;18(1):6–14.

23. Coakley FV, Hricak H. Radiologic anatomy of the prostate gland: a clinical approach. Radiol Clin North Am 2000;38(1):15–30.

24. McNeal JE. The zonal anatomy of the prostate. Prostate 1981;2(1):35–49.

25. Well D, Yang H, Houseni M, et al. Age-related structural and metabolic changes in the pelvic reproductive end organs. Semin Nucl Med 2007;37(3): 173–84.

26. Nunes LW, Schiebler MS, Rauschning W, et al. The normal prostate and periprostatic structures: correlation between MR images made with an endorectal coil and cadaveric microtome sections. AJR Am J Roentgenol 1995;164(4):923–7.

27. Hricak H, Dooms GC, McNeal JE, et al. MR imaging of the prostate gland: normal anatomy. AJR Am J Roentgenol 1987;148(1):51–8.

28. Phillips ME, Kressel HY, Spritzer CE, et al. Normal prostate and adjacent structures: MR imaging at 1.5 T. Radiology 1987;164(2):381–5.

29. Villeirs GM, Lv K, De Neve WJ, et al. Magnetic resonance imaging anatomy of the prostate and periprostatic area: a guide for radiotherapists. Radiother Oncol 2005;76(1):99–106.

30. King BF, Hattery RR, Lieber MM, et al. Seminal vesicle imaging. Radiographics 1989;9(4):653–76.

31. Secaf E, Nuruddin RN, Hricak H, et al. MR imaging of the seminal vesicles. AJR Am J Roentgenol 1991;156(5):989–94.

32. Schnall MD, Pollack HM, Van Arsdalen K, et al. The seminal tract in patients with ejaculatory dysfunction: MR imaging with an endorectal surface coil. AJR Am J Roentgenol 1992;159(2):337–41.

33. Futterer JJ, Heijmink SW, Spermon JR. Imaging the male reproductive tract: current trends and future directions. Radiol Clin North Am 2008;46(1): 133–47, vii.

34. Krieger JN, Riley DE, Cheah PY, et al. Epidemiology of prostatitis: new evidence for a worldwide problem. World J Urol 2003;21(2):70–4.

35. Batstone GR, Doble A. Chronic prostatitis. Curr Opin Urol 2003;13(1):23–9.

36. Lipsky BA. Prostatitis and urinary tract infection in men: what's new; what's true? Am J Med 1999;106(3):327–34.

37. Krieger JN, Lee SW, Jeon J, et al. Epidemiology of prostatitis. Int J Antimicrob Agents 2008;31(Suppl 1):S85–90.

38. Atilla MK, Sargin H, Odabas O, et al. Evaluation of 42 patients with chronic abacterial prostatitis: are there any underlying correctable pathologies? Int Urol Nephrol 1998;30(4):463–9.

39. Maeda H, Toyooka N, Kinukawa T, et al. Magnetic resonance images of hematospermia. Urology 1993;41(5):499–504.

40. Shukla-Dave A, Hricak H, Eberhardt SC, et al. Chronic prostatitis: MR imaging and 1H MR spectroscopic imaging findings—initial observations. Radiology 2004;231(3):717–24.

41. McDermott VG, Meakem TJ 3rd, Stolpen AH, et al. Prostatic and periprostatic cysts: findings on MR imaging. AJR Am J Roentgenol 1995;164(1):123–7.

42. Aalame NM, Sulser T, Egli U, et al. Primary male infertility caused by congenital prostatic cyst: sonographic and magnetic resonance imaging findings. Urol Int 1998;61(1):58–61.

43. Thurnher S, Hricak H, Tanagho EA. Mullerian duct cyst: diagnosis with MR imaging. Radiology 1988;168(1):25–8.

44. Nghiem HT, Kellman GM, Sandberg SA, et al. Cystic lesions of the prostate. Radiographics 1990;10(4):635–50.

45. Parsons RB, Fisher AM, Bar-Chama N, et al. MR imaging in male infertility. Radiographics 1997;17(3):627–37.

46. Littrup PJ, Lee F, McLeary RD, et al. Transrectal US of the seminal vesicles and ejaculatory ducts: clinical correlation. Radiology 1988;168(3):625–8.

47. Robert Y, Rigot JM, Rocourt N, et al. MR findings of ejaculatory duct cysts. Acta Radiol 1994;35(5):459–62.

48. Ogreid P, Hatteland K. Cyst of seminal vesicle associated with ipsilateral renal agenesis. A report on four cases. Scand J Urol Nephrol 1979;13(1):113–6.

49. King BF, Hattery RR, Lieber MM, et al. Congenital cystic disease of the seminal vesicle. Radiology 1991;178(1):207–11.

50. Belet U, Danaci M, Sarikaya S, et al. Prevalence of epididymal, seminal vesicle, prostate, and testicular cysts in autosomal-dominant polycystic kidney disease. Urology 2002;60(1):138–41.

51. Gevenois PA, Van Sinoy ML, Sintzoff SA Jr, et al. Cysts of the prostate and seminal vesicles: MR imaging findings in 11 cases. AJR Am J Roentgenol 1990;155(5):1021–4.

52. Chang YH, Chuang CK, Ng KF, et al. Coexistence of a hemorrhagic cyst and carcinoma in the prostate gland. Chang Gung Med J 2005;28(4):264–7.

53. Papanicolaou N, Pfister RC, Stafford SA, et al. Prostatic abscess: imaging with transrectal sonography and MR. AJR Am J Roentgenol 1987;149(5):981–2.

54. Barozzi L, Pavlica P, Menchi I, et al. Prostatic abscess: diagnosis and treatment. AJR Am J Roentgenol 1998;170(3):753–7.

55. Cytron S, Weinberger M, Pitlik SD, et al. Value of transrectal ultrasonography for diagnosis and treatment of prostatic abscess. Urology 1988;32(5):454–8.

56. Wall SD, Fisher MR, Amparo EG, et al. Magnetic resonance imaging in the evaluation of abscesses. AJR Am J Roentgenol 1985;144(6):1217–21.

57. Patil PS, Elem B. Schistosomiasis of the prostate and the seminal vesicles: observations in Zambia. J Trop Med Hyg 1988;91(5):245–8.

58. Vilana R, Corachan M, Gascon J, et al. Schistosomiasis of the male genital tract: transrectal sonographic findings. J Urol 1997;158(4):1491–3.

59. Schwartz E, Pick N, Shazberg G, et al. Hematospermia due to schistosome infection in travelers: diagnostic and treatment challenges. Clin Infect Dis 2002;35(11):1420–4.

60. McKenna G, Schousboe M, Paltridge G. Subjective change in ejaculate as symptom of infection with Schistosoma haematobium in travelers. BMJ 1997;315(7114):1000–1.

61. Murdoch DR. Hematospermia due to schistosome infection in travelers. Clin Infect Dis 2003;36(8):1086.

62. Corachan M, Valls ME, Gascon J, et al. Hematospermia: a new etiology of clinical interest. Am J Trop Med Hyg 1994;50(5):580–4.

63. Premkumar A, Newhouse JH. Seminal vesicle tuberculosis: CT appearance. J Comput Assist Tomogr 1988;12(4):676–7.

64. Wang JH, Chang T. Tuberculosis of the prostate: CT appearance. J Comput Assist Tomogr 1991;15(2):269–70.

65. Das KM, Indudhara R, Vaidyanathan S. Sonographic features of genitourinary tuberculosis. AJR Am J Roentgenol 1992;158(2):327–9.

66. Tajima H, Tajima N, Hiraoka Y, et al. Tuberculosis of the prostate: MR imaging. Radiat Med 1995;13(4):171–3.

67. Wang LJ, Wong YC, Chen CJ, et al. CT features of genitourinary tuberculosis. J Comput Assist Tomogr 1997;21(2):254–8.

68. Wang JH, Sheu MH, Lee RC. Tuberculosis of the prostate: MR appearance. J Comput Assist Tomogr 1997;21(4):639–40.

69. Lawrentschuk N, Pan D, Stillwell R, et al. Implications of amyloidosis on prostatic biopsy. Int J Urol 2004;11(10):925–7.

70. Singh SK, Wadhwa P, Nada R, et al. Localized primary amyloidosis of the prostate, bladder, and ureters. Int J Urol Nephrol 2005;37(3):495–7.

71. Wilson SK, Buchanan RD, Stone WJ, et al. J Urol 1973 Sep;110(3):322–3.

72. Orland SM, Hanno PM, Wein AJ. Prostatitis, prostatosis, and prostatodynia. Urology 1985;25(5):439–59.

73. Mulhall JP, Albertsen PC. Hemospermia: diagnosis and management. Urology 1995;46(4):463–7.

74. Leary FJ, Aguilo JJ. Clinical significance of hematospermia. Mayo Clin Proc 1974;49(11):815–7.

75. Leary FJ. Hematospermia. J Fam Pract 1975;2(3):185–6.

76. Han M, Brannigan RE, Antenor JA, et al. Association of hemospermia with prostate cancer. J Urol 2004;172(6 Pt 1 of 2):2189–92.

77. Lencioni R, Ortori S, Cioni D, et al. Endorectal coil MR imaging findings in hemospermia. MAGMA 1999;8(2):91–7.

78. Cho IR, Lee MS, Rha KH, et al. Magnetic resonance imaging in hemospermia. J Urol 1997;157(1):258–62.

79. Mazhar D, Waxman J. Prostate cancer. Postgrad Med J 2002;78(924):590–5.

80. Walsh PC. Surgery and the reduction of mortality from prostate cancer. N Engl J Med 2002;347(11):839–40.

81. Jemal A, Siegel R, Ward E, et al. Cancer statistics, 2008. CA Cancer J Clin 2008;58(2):71–96.

82. Michaelson MD, Cotter SE, Gargollo PC, et al. Management of complications of prostate cancer treatment. CA Cancer J Clin 2008;58(4):196–213.

83. Young JL Jr, Percy CL, Asire AJ, et al. Cancer incidence and mortality in the United States, 1973–77. Natl Cancer Inst Monogr 1981;(57):1–187.

84. Mitka M. Disparity in cancer statistics changing. JAMA 2002;287(6):703–4.

85. Ikonen S, Kivisaari L, Tervahartiala P, et al. Prostatic MR imaging. Accuracy in differentiating cancer from other prostatic disorders. Acta Radiol 2001;42(4):348–54.

86. Li H, Sugimura K, Kaji Y, et al. Conventional MRI capabilities in the diagnosis of prostate cancer in the transition zone. AJR Am J Roentgenol 2006;186(3):729–42.

87. McNeal J, Noldus J. Limitations of transition zone needle biopsy findings in the prediction of transition zone cancer and tissue composition of benign nodular hyperplasia. Urology 1996;48(5):751–6.

88. Carrol CL, Sommer FG, McNeal JE, et al. The abnormal prostate: MR imaging at 1.5 T with histopathologic correlation. Radiology 1987;163(2):521–5.

89. Hricak H, Dooms GC, Jeffrey RB, et al. Prostatic carcinoma: staging by clinical assessment, CT, and MR imaging. Radiology 1987;162(2):331–6.

90. Schnall MD, Imai Y, Tomaszewski J, et al. Prostate cancer: local staging with endorectal surface coil MR imaging. Radiology 1991;178(3):797–802.

91. Schiebler ML, Schnall MD, Pollack HM, et al. Current role of MR imaging in the staging of adenocarcinoma of the prostate. Radiology 1993;189(2):339–52.

92. Schnall MD, Bezzi M, Pollack HM, et al. Magnetic resonance imaging of the prostate. Magn Reson Q 1990;6(1):1–16.

93. Yu KK, Hricak H, Alagappan R, et al. Detection of extracapsular extension of prostate carcinoma with endorectal and phased-array coil MR imaging: multivariate feature analysis. Radiology 1997;202(3):697–702.

94. Macura KJ. Multiparametric magnetic resonance imaging of the prostate: current status in prostate cancer detection, localization, and staging. Semin Roentgenol 2008;43(4):303–13.

95. Schnall MD, Pollack HM. Magnetic resonance imaging of the prostate gland. Urol Radiol 1990;12(2):109–14.

96. Schiebler ML, Yankaskas BC, Tempany C, et al. MR imaging in adenocarcinoma of the prostate: interobserver variation and efficacy for determining stage C disease. AJR Am J Roentgenol 1992;158(3):559–62 [discussion: 63–4].

97. Outwater EK, Petersen RO, Siegelman ES, et al. Prostate carcinoma: assessment of diagnostic criteria for capsular penetration on endorectal coil MR images. Radiology 1994;193(2):333–9.

98. Bernstein MR, Cangiano T, D'Amico A, et al. Endorectal coil magnetic resonance imaging and clinicopathologic findings in T1c adenocarcinoma of the prostate. Urol Oncol 2000;5(3):104–7.

99. May F, Treumann T, Dettmar P, et al. Limited value of endorectal magnetic resonance imaging and transrectal ultrasonography in the staging of clinically localized prostate cancer. BJU Int 2001;87(1):66–9.

100. Cornud F, Flam T, Chauveinc L, et al. Extraprostatic spread of clinically localized prostate cancer: factors predictive of pT3 tumor and of positive endorectal MR imaging examination results. Radiology 2002;224(1):203–10.

101. Bloch BN, Furman-Haran E, Helbich TH, et al. Prostate cancer: accurate determination of extracapsular extension with high spatial resolution dynamic contrast-enhanced and T2-weighted MR imaging—initial results. Radiology 2007;245(1):176–85.

102. Akin O, Sala E, Moskowitz CS, et al. Transition zone prostate cancers: features, detection, localization, and staging at endorectal MR imaging. Radiology 2006;239(3):784–92.

103. Seitz M, Shukla-Dave A, Bjartell A, et al. Functional magnetic resonance imaging in prostate cancer. Eur Urol 2009;55(4):801–14.

104. Masterson TA, Touijer K. The role of endorectal coil MRI in preoperative staging and decision making

for the treatment of clinically localized prostate cancer. MAGMA 2008;21(6):371–7.

105. Hersh MR, Knapp EL, Choi J. Newer imaging modalities to assess tumor in the prostate. Cancer Control 2004;11(6):353–7.

106. Wefer AE, Hricak H, Vigneron DB, et al. Sextant localization of prostate cancer: comparison of sextant biopsy, magnetic resonance imaging, and magnetic resonance spectroscopic imaging with step section histology. J Urol 2000;164(2):400–4.

107. Hasumi M, Suzuki K, Taketomi A, et al. The combination of multivoxel MR spectroscopy with MR imaging improve the diagnostic accuracy for localization of prostate cancer. Anticancer Res 2003;23(5b):4223–7.

108. Portalez D, Malavaud B, Herigault G, et al. [Predicting prostate cancer with dynamic endorectal coil MR and proton spectroscopic MR imaging] [in French]. J Radiol 2004;85(12 Pt 1):1999–2004.

109. Squillaci E, Manenti G, Mancino S, et al. MR spectroscopy of prostate cancer. Initial clinical experience. J Exp Clin Cancer Res 2005;24(4):523–30.

110. Vilanova JC, Barcelo J. Prostate cancer detection: magnetic resonance (MR) spectroscopic imaging. Abdom Imaging 2007;32(2):253–61.

111. Yu KK, Scheidler J, Hricak H, et al. Prostate cancer: prediction of extracapsular extension with endorectal MR imaging and three-dimensional proton MR spectroscopic imaging. Radiology 1999;213(2):481–8.

112. Wang L, Hricak H, Kattan MW, et al. Prediction of organ-confined prostate cancer: incremental value of MR imaging and MR spectroscopic imaging to staging nomograms. Radiology 2006;238(2):597–603.

113. Zakian KL, Sircar K, Hricak H, et al. Correlation of proton MR spectroscopic imaging with gleason score based on step section pathologic analysis after radical prostatectomy. Radiology 2005;234(3):804–14.

114. Weinreb JC, Blume JD, Coakley FV, et al. Prostate cancer: sextant localization at MR imaging and MR spectroscopic imaging before prostatectomy—results of ACRIN prospective multi-institutional clinicopathologic study. Radiology 2009;251(1):122–33.

115. Morgan VA, Kyriazi S, Ashley SE, et al. Evaluation of the potential of diffusion-weighted imaging in prostate cancer detection. Acta Radiol 2007;48(6):695–703.

116. Torigian DA, Huang SS, Houseni M, et al. Functional imaging of cancer with emphasis on molecular techniques. CA Cancer J Clin 2007;57(4):206–24.

117. Futterer JJ, Heijmink SW, Scheenen TW, et al. Prostate cancer localization with dynamic contrast-enhanced MR imaging and proton MR spectroscopic imaging. Radiology 2006;241(2):449–58.

118. Barentsz JO, Futterer JJ, Takahashi S. Use of ultra-small superparamagnetic iron oxide in lymph node MR imaging in prostate cancer patients. Eur J Radiol 2007;63(3):369–72.

119. Messing EM, Manola J, Sarosdy M, et al. Immediate hormonal therapy compared with observation after radical prostatectomy and pelvic lymphadenectomy in men with node-positive prostate cancer. N Engl J Med 1999;341(24):1781–8.

120. Harisinghani MG, Barentsz J, Hahn PF, et al. Noninvasive detection of clinically occult lymph node metastases in prostate cancer. N Engl J Med 2003;348(25):2491–9.

121. Carmel M, Masse SR, Lehoux JG, et al. Leiomyosarcoma of prostate. Urology 1983;22(2):190–3.

122. Bartolozzi C, Selli C, Olmastroni M, et al. Rhabdomyosarcoma of the prostate: MR findings. AJR Am J Roentgenol 1988;150(6):1333–4.

123. Russo P, Demas B, Reuter V. Adult prostatic sarcoma. Abdom Imaging 1993;18(4):399–401.

124. Gaudin PB, Rosai J, Epstein JI. Sarcomas and related proliferative lesions of specialized prostatic stroma: a clinicopathologic study of 22 cases. Am J Surg Pathol 1998;22(2):148–62.

125. Varghese SL, Grossfeld GD. The prostatic gland: malignancies other than adenocarcinomas. Radiol Clin North Am 2000;38(1):179–202.

126. Sexton WJ, Lance RE, Reyes AO, et al. Adult prostate sarcoma: the M.D. Anderson Cancer Center experience. J Urol 2001;166(2):521–5.

FDG PET in Prostate Cancer

Hossein Jadvar, MD, PhD, MPH, MBA*

KEYWORDS
- PET • CT • FDG • Prostate • Cancer

The role of positron emission tomography (PET) with [F-18]-fluorodeoxyglucose (FDG) for the imaging evaluation of patients who have cancer has expanded rapidly worldwide. The increasing use of FDG-PET and PET-CT in cancer imaging have been facilitated by the development of hybrid PET-CT imaging systems that can precisely localize metabolic abnormalities and characterize the metabolic activity of normal and abnormal structures; commercial regional distribution of FDG; growing clinical experience, recently spearheaded by National Oncologic PET Registry (NOPR; http://www.cancerPETregistry.org/); and improved understanding of clinical indications and reimbursement. FDG-PET has been used for diagnosis, initial staging, restaging, prediction, and monitoring of treatment response, surveillance, and prognostication in various cancers, and leads to improved clinical decision making and cost-effective management changes in a considerable number of patients.[1–3]

The exact clinical use of PET and PET-CT in prostate cancer is currently being explored. The recent publications summarizing the NOPR findings showed that prostate cancer was one of the most common cancers with patient enrollment.[4,5] This article first reviews the limited available data on the molecular biology basis of FDG accumulation in prostate cancer, and then briefly reviews the current clinical experience with the use of PET with FDG in the imaging evaluation of prostate cancer.

GLUCOSE METABOLISM IN PROSTATE CANCER

Several hallmarks of cancer have been described that include self-sufficiency in growth signals, insensitivity to antigrowth signals, evasion of apoptosis, limitless replicative potential, sustained angiogenesis, tissue invasion and launch of metastasis envoys, evasion of tumors from the immune system, and increased glucose metabolism.[6,7] The ability of FDG-PET to detect cancer is based on the latter hallmark (Warburg effect). The relationship between tumor growth and the inefficient energy production from glucose metabolism is not well understood but may be explained in terms of adaptation to hypoxia through up-regulation of glucose transporters and increased enzymatic activity of hexokinase.[8,9]

Glucose transporter (GLUTx, although the currently approved gene symbol is SLC2Ax) is the first rate-limiting step for glucose metabolism that allows energy-independent glucose transport across the cell membrane down the concentration gradient while hexokinase-II phosphorylates glucose to glucose-6-phosphate. Similarly, FDG is phosphorylated to FDG-6-phosphate but, contrary to glucose-6-phosphate, cannot be metabolized further in the glycolytic pathway and becomes trapped in the cell because of its negative charge and the very low activity of the reverse enzyme, glucose-6-phophatase, in most cancers.[10–15]

GLUT1 mRNA expression has been assessed in the androgen-independent cell lines DU145 and PC-3, and the androgen-sensitive cell line LNCaP.[16] The poorly differentiated androgen-independent cell lines showed higher mRNA expression than the well-differentiated androgen-sensitive cell line, suggesting that GLUT1 expression is directly related to the malignancy grade. One study evaluated the expression of several hypoxia-associated genes within benign prostatic

This work was supported by National Institutes of Health–National Cancer Institute grant no. R01-CA111613.
* Division of Nuclear Medicine, Department of Radiology, Keck School of Medicine, University of Southern California, 2250 Alcazar Street, CSC 102, Los Angeles, CA 90033, USA
E-mail address: jadvar@usc.edu

PET Clin 4 (2009) 155–161
doi:10.1016/j.cpet.2009.05.002

hyperplasia (BPH) and human prostate cancer tissue (Gleason score, 5–10).[17] GLUT1 gene expression was not only significantly higher in the tumor than in BPH but also correlated directly with Gleason score (R = 0.274; P = .026), corroborating the direct relationship between GLUT1 expression and tumor grade.

Other in vitro studies have also shown that FDG uptake increases with hypoxic condition in androgen-sensitive and -independent prostate cancer cell lines.[18] Moreover, hypoxia resulted in up-regulation of hypoxia-inducible factors HIF-1α and HIF-2α that could be inhibited with the nonsteroidal anti-inflammatory drug ibuprofen, leading to cyclooxygenase-2–independent down-regulation of the HIF-regulated proteins vascular endothelial growth factor and GLUT1.[19]

The glucose metabolism of prostate cancer may not be limited to GLUT1, because another investigation showed that GLUT12 may also be involved.[20] The modulatory effect of androgen on tumor glucose metabolism has also been investigated. Higher FDG accumulation has been observed in androgen-independent tumors than in those that are androgen-sensitive.[21] Accordingly, castration has been observed to reduce glucose metabolism in the prostate tumor.[21–23]

In summary, despite limited data, glucose metabolism in prostate cancer seems to be GLUT-mediated, but the relationship is complex and may be affected by many factors, such as hypoxia and androgen level.

CLINICAL USE OF FDG-PET IN PROSTATE CANCER

Considerable heterogeneity exists in the current clinical experience with FDG-PET in prostate cancer, because of variability in disease states, validation criteria, and end points among studies.[24–26] Additional complicating factors include the inherent biologic and clinical heterogeneity of the disease, and technical and image processing factors (eg, filtered-back projection compared with iterative reconstruction with segmented attenuation) irrespective of the underlying biologic heterogeneity.[18,27–29]

Normal Prostate

The authors recently reported on the FDG accumulation in the normal prostate gland in relation to age and prostate size in PET-CT studies performed on 145 men (age range, 22–97 years) who had no clinical and laboratory evidence of prostate pathology.[30] The population average and range of the normal prostate size were 4.3 ± 0.5 cm (mean ± SD) and 2.9 to 5.5 cm,

respectively. The population average of mean and maximum standardized uptake value (SUV, as semi-quantitative measure of the amount of tracer accumulation in a region of interest normalized to body weight and injected tracer dose) was 1.3 ± 0.4 (range, 0.1–2.7) and 1.6 ± 0.4 (range, 1.1–3.7), respectively. Mean SUV tended to decrease as the prostate size increased (r = −0.16; P = .058), whereas the prostate tended to get larger as age increased (r = 0.32; P<.001). Despite the generally low FDG uptake by the normal prostate gland, however, other studies have shown that significant overlap can exist among FDG accumulation in normal prostate, BPH, and prostate cancer.[25,26,31–34]

Diagnosis and Initial Staging

FDG-PET may not be useful in diagnosing and staging clinically organ-confined disease and detecting locally recurrent disease, because of overlap of tumor uptake with scar tissue and the obscuring that can occur from intense urine activity in the adjacent urinary bladder.[32,35] FDG is also not specific for cancer, and false-positives may occur with inflammatory condition such as prostatitis.[36]

However, despite these less-enthusiastic observations, several animal-based translational and human-based clinical studies have shown that FDG-PET can be useful in specific clinical circumstances in prostate cancer. FDG uptake in prostate cancer increases directly with increasing Gleason grade, clinical stage, and serum prostate-specific antigen (PSA) level.[37,38] In an early experience with 34 men who had prostate cancer and known or suspected metastatic disease, FDG-PET showed an SUV range of 2.1 to 5.7 for the metastatic lesions, with the notation that PET was less sensitive than bone scintigraphy and detection of pelvic lymph node metastases was limited because of intense bladder urine activity.[39] However, in patients who had known osseous metastatic disease, FDG-PET may distinguish the metabolically active lesions from the metabolically quiescent lesions.[40–42] Also, recent data from the authors' laboratory suggest that FDG-PET concordance rate with other imaging studies seems to be higher in the castrate-resistant disease than the castrate-sensitive disease, and also higher for lymph nodes and visceral lesions than for osseous lesions.[43]

Prostate-Specific Antigen Relapse Only

A large group of men present with "PSA relapse only" (biochemical failure) at some point after definitive therapy, who by definition have no standard imaging evidence of disease. In this group of men, "nonstandard" imaging detection of disease can direct appropriate treatment, such as salvage radiation therapy for local recurrence in the prostate bed or systemic therapy for metastatic disease (**Figs. 1** and **2**).

In one study of 24 patients who had a rising serum PSA level after treatment for localized prostate cancer, FDG-PET was performed before pelvic lymph node dissection.[44] In accordance with PSA relapse only disease, all men had negative findings on whole-body bone scan and equivocal pelvic CT results. Validation was achieved through histology of the pelvic lymph nodes harvested at surgery in 67% of patients. The authors reported a sensitivity of 75%, specificity of 100%, accuracy of 83.3%, positive predictive value of 100%, and negative predictive value of 67.7% in detecting metastatic pelvic lymph nodes in this relatively homogeneous state of disease.

In a similar investigation of 91 patients who had PSA relapse after prostatectomy, validated with biopsy or clinical and imaging follow-up, the researchers reported that mean PSA level was higher in patients who had positive PET results than in those whose results were negative (9.5 ± 2.2 versus 2.1 ± 3.3 ng/mL).[45] Using a receiver operating characteristic curve analysis, the best tradeoff between sensitivity and specificity was found at a PSA level of 2.4 ng/mL (80%, 73%, respectively) and PSA velocity of 1.3 ng/mL per year (71%, 77%, respectively). The authors reported that FDG-PET detected local or systemic disease in 31% of patients who experienced PSA relapse. However, confidence in the accuracy and relevance of this figure is guarded, given the

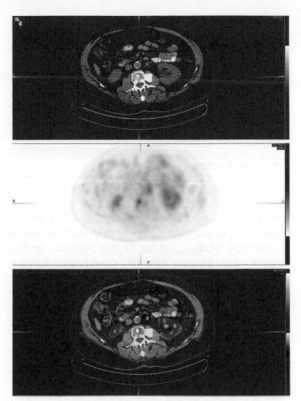

Fig. 2. Axial CT (*top panel*), [F-18]-fluorodeoxyglucose (FDG) positron emission tomography (FDG-PET) (*middle panel*), and fused PET-CT (*bottom panel*) of metastatic prostate cancer involving L2 vertebral body (maximum standardized uptake value [SUVmax] = 4.8) and a conglomerate of subcentimeter left para-aortic nodes (SUVmax = 3.3; largest single node, 9 mm).

definition of PSA relapse and the heterogeneity of the validation criteria, frequent with other similar studies.[46] Other studies have shown that FDG-PET may be particularly useful in men who have a rising PSA level despite treatment and that, in the clinical setting of PSA relapse, it is more sensitive than indium-111–capromab pendetide scintigraphy.[47,48]

Evaluation of Treatment Response

FDG-PET was also investigated for its use in assessing response to treatment. An earlier prostate cancer study in rats was disappointing, showing that the global FDG uptake was unchanged after treatment with gemcitabine.[49] However, a later investigation showed that FDG accumulation in the primary prostate cancer and metastatic sites decreased 1 to 5 months after initiation of androgen-deprivation therapy, similar

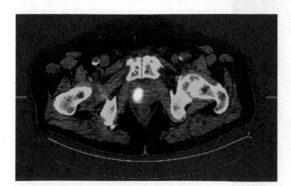

Fig. 1. Axial fused [F-18]-fluorodeoxyglucose positron emission tomography/CT of locally recurrent disease in right prostate lobe 11 years after radiation therapy for primary moderately differentiated prostate cancer with Gleason sum score of 4.

in principle to the results of the animal xenograft studies.[21,50,51]

The authors' preliminary results with androgen deprivation and various chemotherapy regimens have shown that the tumor accumulation of FDG uptake decreases with successful treatment in concordance with other measures of response, such as decline in serum PSA level (**Fig. 3**).

Prognostication

Studies have also shown that the level and extent of FDG accumulation in metastatic lesions may also provide information on prognosis. One investigation reported that a greater than 33% increase in average SUV_{max} of up to five lesions, or the appearance of new lesions, could dichotomize patients who have castrate metastatic prostate cancer treated with antimicrotubule chemotherapy as either progressors or non-progressors.[52] Similar prognostic use was shown, in that men who had highly FDG-avid primary prostate tumors had a poorer prognosis compared with those who had low SUV.[53]

Because FDG uptake in the prostate tumor seems to be initially dependent on androgen, FDG-PET may also be useful in predicting the time-to-androgen–refractory state (eg, early increase in tumor FDG uptake during castrate state) that may allow an early intervention to avert or delay this clinical state and improve overall patient outcome.[21]

National Oncologic PET Registry and Prostate Cancer

The NOPR was established in May 2006 to collect and analyze data on the clinical use of FDG-PET to provide evidence for reimbursement coverage by the Centers for Medicare & Medicaid Services.[4] The results were recently reported for the first 2 years of data from 40,863 PET scans for staging, restaging, or detection of suspected recurrence in patients who had pathologically proven cancers.[5] The most number of FDG-PET scans (5309 scans, equivalent to 13% of all scans) was performed in patients who had prostate cancer.

PET findings changed clinical management in 35.1% of prostate cancer cases (95% CI, 33.8%–36.4%), although the odds ratio for change in management compared with that for other cancers in the NOPR trial was less than 1 (0.86; 95% CI, 0.81–0.92), implying that chance of management change was lower for prostate cancer than for all other cancer types. The change in management was from non-treatment to treatment in 25.3% and from treatment to non-treatment in 9.7% of cases, with a major change in type of treatment relative to the plan before PET in 8.5% of cases. The PET-directed change in management was nearly equal in relation to the testing indications, with 32.0% (30.0%–34.1%) for initial staging (n = 2042 cases), 34.0% (95% CI, 31.6%–36.4%) for restaging (n = 1477 cases), and 39.4% (95% CI, 37.2%–41.7%) for detection of suspected recurrence (n = 1790 cases).

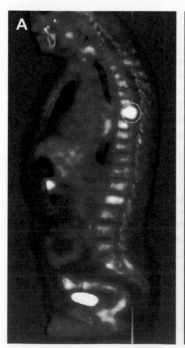 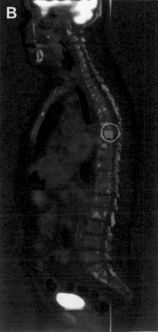

Fig. 3. Sagittal fused [F-18]-fluorodeoxyglucose positron emission tomography/CT in a man with castrate-sensitive metastatic prostate cancer before (*A*) and 5 months after (*B*) androgen-deprivation therapy. Note the decline in the hypermetabolic activity of the sclerotic mid-thoracic spine vertebral body in response to therapy. Lesion maximum standardized uptake value declined from 5.0 before therapy to 2.7 after therapy, corresponding to serum prostate-specific antigen decline from 98 to 21 ng/mL, respectively.

SUMMARY

The current clinical experience with FDG-PET in prostate cancer is afflicted by considerable variability in disease states, validation criteria, and end points. Despite this significant limitation, however, FDG-PET seems to be useful for diagnosing and staging known or suspected primary tumors with high Gleason score; in detecting locally recurrent or metastatic disease in some patients who have PSA relapse only with scan sensitivity that increases with increasing PSA level; in assessing the extent of metabolically active castrate-resistant disease; in monitoring response to androgen deprivation and other therapies; and in prognostication.

As suggested by NOPR trial, FDG-PET can impact the clinical management of men who have prostate cancer, although this impact may be lower than that for other cancers. FDG-PET may be limited in diagnosing and staging clinically organ-confined disease and can be falsely negative because of overlap of tumor uptake with normal, BPH, and scar tissue, and may be falsely positive because of inflammatory conditions. More extensive experience obtained through well-designed clinical trials based on well-defined clinical states of disease and hard end points will help determine the exact role of FDG-PET in prostate cancer. A prospective clinical trial is underway to help define the role of FDG-PET/CT in therapy assessment and in outcome prediction (time-to-hormone– refractory state and survival) in men who have androgen-naïve and -refractory metastatic prostate cancer.[54]

REFERENCES

1. Phelps ME. PET: the merging of biology and imaging into molecular imaging. J Nucl Med 2000;41:661–81.
2. Gambhir SS. Molecular imaging of cancer with positron emission tomography. Nat Rev Cancer 2002;2: 683–93.
3. Basu S, Alavi A. Unparalleled contribution of 18F-FDG PET to medicine over 3 decades. J Nucl Med 2008;49:17N–21N, 37N.
4. Hillner BE, Siegel BA, Liu D, et al. Impact of positron emission tomography/computed tomography and positron mission tomography (PET) alone on expected management of patients with cancer: initial results from the National Oncologic PET Registry. J Clin Oncol 2008;26:4229.
5. Hillner BE, Siegel BA, Shields AF, et al. Relationship between cancer type and impact of PET and PET/CT on intended management: findings of the National Oncologic PET Registry. J Nucl Med 2008;49:1928–35.
6. Hanahan D, Weinberg RA. The hallmarks of cancer. Cell 2000;100:57–70.
7. Gambhir SS. Molecular imaging of cancer: from molecules to humans. Introduction. J Nucl Med 2008;49(Suppl 2):1S–4S.
8. Gillies RJ, Robey I, Gatenby RA. Causes and consequences of increased glucose metabolism of cancers. J Nucl Med 2008;49(6 Suppl):24S–42S.
9. Plathow C, Weber WA. Tumor cell metabolism imaging. J Nucl Med 2008;49(6 Suppl):43S–63S.
10. Medina RA, Owen GI. Glucose transporters: expression, regulation and cancer. Biol Res 2002;35:9–26.
11. Smith TA. Facilitative glucose transporter expression in human cancer tissue. Br J Biomed Sci 1999;56: 285–92.
12. Macheda ML, Rogers S, Bets JD. Molecular and cellular regulation of glucose transport (GLUT) proteins in cancer. J Cell Physiol 2005;202:654–62.
13. Wilson JE. Isoenzymes of mammalian hexokinase: structure, subcellular localization and metabolic function. J Exp Biol 2003;206(Pt 12):2049–57.
14. Smith TA. Mammalian hexokinases and their abnormal expression in cancer. Br J Biomed Sci 2000;57:170–8.
15. Pastorino JG, Hoek JB. Hexokinase II: the integration of energy metabolism and control of apoptosis. Curr Med Chem 2003;10:1535–51.
16. Effert P, Beniers AJ, Tamimi Y, et al. Expression of glucose transporter 1 (GLUT-1) in cell lines and clinical specimen from human prostate adenocarcinoma. Anticancer Res 2004;24(5A):3057–63.
17. Stewardt GD, Gray K, Pennington CJ, et al. Analysis of hypoxia-associated gene expression in prostate cancer: lysyl oxidase and glucose transporter 1 expression correlate with Gleason score. Oncol Rep 2008;20:1561–7.
18. Hara T, Bansal A, DeGrado TR. Effect of hypoxia on the uptake of [methyl-3H]choline, [1-14C]acetate and [18F]FDG in cultured prostate cancer cells. Nucl Med Biol 2006;33:977–84.
19. Palayoor ST, Tofilon PJ, Coleman CN. Ibuprofen-mediated reduction of hypoxia-inducible factors HIF-1alpha and HIF-2alpha in prostate cancer cells. Clin Cancer Res 2003;9:3150–7.
20. Chandler JD, Williams ED, Slavin JL, et al. Expression and localization of GLUT1 and GLUT12 in prostate carcinoma. Cancer 2003;97:2035–42.
21. Jadvar H, Li X, Shahinian A, et al. Glucose metabolism of human prostate cancer mouse xenografts. Mol Imaging 2005;4:91–7.
22. Oyama N, Kim J, Jones LA, et al. MicroPET assessment of androgenic control of glucose and acetate uptake in the rat prostate and a prostate cancer tumor model. Nucl Med Biol 2002;29:783–90.
23. Agus DB, Golde DW, Squouros G, et al. Positron emission tomography of a human prostate cancer xenograft: association of changes in deoxyglucose

accumulation with other measures of outcome following androgen withdrawal. Cancer Res 1998; 58:3009–14.

24. Apolo AB, Pandit-Taskar N, Morris MJ. Novel tracers and their development for the imaging of metastatic prostate cancer. J Nucl Med 2008;49: 2031–41.

25. Takahashi N, Inoue T, Lee J, et al. The roles of PET and PET/CT in the diagnosis and management of prostate cancer. Oncology 2007;72:226–33.

26. Salminen E, Hogg A, Binns D, et al. Investigations with FDG-PET scanning in prostate cancer show limited value for clinical practice. Acta Oncol 2002; 41(5):425–9.

27. Pugachev A, Ruan S, Carlin S, et al. Dependence of FDG uptake on tumor microenvironment. Int J Radiat Oncol Biol Phys 2005;62:545–53.

28. Etchebehere EC, Macapinlac HA, Gonen M, et al. Qualitative and quantitative comparison between images obtained with filtered back projection and iterative reconstruction in prostate cancer lesions of 18F-FDG PET. Q J Nucl Med 2002;46: 122–30.

29. Turlakow A, Larson SM, Coakley F, et al. Local detection of prostate cancer by positron emission tomography with 2-fluorodeoxyglucose: comparison of filtered back projection and iterative reconstruction with segmented attenuation correction. Q J Nucl Med 2001;45:235–44.

30. Jadvar H, Ye W, Groshen S, et al. [F-8]-fluorodeoxyglucose PET-CT of the normal prostate gland. Ann Nucl Med 2008;22:787–93.

31. Effert PJ, Bares R, Handt S, et al. Metabolic imaging of untreated prostate cancer by positron emission tomography with 18fluorine-labeled deoxyglucose. J Urol 1996;155:994–8.

32. Hofer C, Laubenbacher C, Block T, et al. Fluorine-18-fluorodeoxyglucose positron emission tomography is useless for the detection of local recurrence after radical prostatectomy. Eur Urol 1999;36:31–5.

33. Patel P, Cohade C, DeWeese T, et al. Evaluation of metabolic activity of prostate gland with PET-CT. J Nucl Med 2002;43(5 Suppl):119P.

34. von Mallek D, Backhaus B, Muller SC, et al. Technical limits of PET/CT with 18FDG in prostate cancer. Aktuelle Urol 2006;37:218–21.

35. Liu IJ, Zafar MB, Lai YH, et al. Fluorodeoxyglucose positron emission tomography studies in diagnosis and staging of clinically organ-confined prostate cancer. Urology 2001;57:108–11.

36. Kao PF, Chou YH, Iai CW. Diffuse FDG uptake in acute prostatitis. Clin Nucl Med 2008;33:308–10.

37. Oyama N, Akino H, Suzuki Y, et al. The increased accumulation of [18F]fluorodeoxyglucose in untreated prostate cancer. Jpn J Clin Oncol 1999;29: 623–0.

38. Kanamaru H, Oyama N, Akino H, et al. Evaluation of prostate cancer using FDG-PET. Hinyokika Kiyo 2000;46:851–3.

39. Shreve PD, Grossman HB, Gross MD, et al. Metastatic prostate cancer: initial findings of PET with FDG. Radiology 1996;199:751–6.

40. Morris NJ, Akhurst T, Osman I, et al. Fluorinated deoxyglucose positron emission tomography imaging in progressive metastatic prostate cancer. Urology 2002;59:913–8.

41. Yeh SD, Imbriaco M, Larson SM, et al. Detection of bony metastases of androgen-independent prostate cancer by PET-FDG. Nucl Med Biol 1996;23:693–7.

42. Jadvar H, Pinski J, Conti P. FDG PET in suspected recurrent and metastatic prostate cancer. Oncol Rep 2003;10(5):1485–8.

43. Jadvar H, Pinski J, Quinn D, et al. Concordance among FDG PET, CT and bone scan in men with metastatic prostate cancer. Proceedings of SNM 55th Annual Meeting, New Orleans (LA): 2008. p. 373P.

44. Chang CH, Wu HC, Tsai JJ, et al. Detecting metastatic pelvic lymph nodes by (18)f-2-deoxyglucose positron emission tomography in patients with prostate-specific antigen relapse after treatment for localized prostate cancer. Urol Int 2003;70(4): 311–5.

45. Schoder H, Herrmann K, Gonen M, et al. 2-[18F]fluoro-2-deoxyglucose positron emission tomography for detection of disease in patients with prostate-specific antigen relapse after radical prostatectomy. Clin Cancer Res 2005;11:4761–9.

46. Sanz G, Robles JE, Gimenez M, et al. Positron emission tomography with 18fluorine-labelled deoxyglucose: utility in localized and advanced prostate cancer. BJU Int 1999;84:1028–31.

47. Sung J, Espiritu JI, Segall GM, et al. Fluorodeoxyglucose positron emission tomography studies in the diagnosis and staging of clinically advanced prostate cancer. BJU Int 2003;92:24–7.

48. Seltzer MA, Barbaric Z, Belldegrun A, et al. Comparison of helical computerized tomography, positron emission tomography and monoclonal antibody scans for evaluation of lymph node metastases in patients with prostate specific antigen relapse after treatment for localized prostate cancer. J Urol 1999;162:1322–8.

49. Haberkorn U, Bellemann ME, Altmann A, et al. PET 2-fluoro-2-deoxyglucose uptake in rat prostate adenocarcinoma during chemotherapy with gemcitabine. J Nucl Med 1997;38:1215–21.

50. Oyama N, Akino H, Suzuki Y, et al. FDG PET for evaluating the change of glucose metabolism in prostate cancer after androgen ablation. Nucl Med Commun 2001;22:963–9.

51. Zhang Y, Saylor M, Wen S, et al. Longitudinally quantitative 2-deoxy-2-[18F]fluoro-D-glucose micro positron emission tomography imaging for efficacy of new anticancer drugs: a case study with bortezomib in prostate cancer murine model. Mol Imaging Biol 2006;8:300–8.

52. Morris MJ, Akhurst T, Larson SM, et al. Fluorodeoxyglucose positron emission tomography as an outcome measure for castrate metastatic prostate cancer treated with antimicrotubule chemotherapy. Clin Cancer Res 2005;11:3210–6.

53. Oyama N, Akino H, Suzuki Y, et al. Prognostic value of 2-deoxy-2-[F-18]fluoro-D-glucose positron emission tomography imaging for patients with prostate cancer. Mol Imaging Biol 2002;4:99–104.

54. Jadvar H. [F-18]-fluorodeoxyglucose (FDG) positron emission tomography and computed tomography (PET-CT) in metastatic prostate cancer. USC Norris Comprehensive Cancer Center. Available at: http://www.clinicaltrials.gov/ct2/show/NCT00282906. Accessed June 17, 2009.

PET Imaging of Prostate Cancer Using ^{11}C-Acetate

Johannes Czernin, MD*, Matthias R. Benz, MD,
Martin S. Allen-Auerbach, MD

KEYWORDS

- Prostate cancer • PET • ^{11}C-Acetate
- Detection • Bio-distribution • Pharmacokinetics
- Protocols • Pathways

Tumor metabolic imaging has focused largely on the use of positron emission tomography (PET) with ^{18}F-fluorodeoxyglucose (FDG), because many cancers are highly glycolytic even in aerobic conditions.[1] However, some cancers do not consistently exhibit increased FDG uptake, and therefore imaging of other metabolic pathways, such as amino acid or lipid metabolism, has been explored in cancer.[2] Prostate cancer exhibits increased glycolysis frequently only in late stages of the disease. However, several studies have shown that lipid metabolism is increased even in early stages of the disease. The lipogenic phenotype of prostate cancer can be imaged, among others, with ^{11}C-acetate PET.

In the 2007 "Cancer Trends Progress Report," the National Cancer Institute reported 165 new cases of prostate cancer per 100,000 men per year. The lifetime chance for developing prostate cancer is approximately 15%, with the cancer risk increasing sharply with age.

EARLY DETECTION

Early detection of initial and recurrent disease is critical for improving patient outcomes. Prostate cancer is usually detected with serum measurements of prostate specific antigen (PSA) or digital rectal examination. Both have a limited sensitivity and specificity.[3] Transrectal ultrasound, although also used for disease detection, is most frequently used for guiding prostate core biopsies in patients who have elevated PSA or abnormal findings on digital rectal examination. However, this imaging approach does not detect disease when PSA levels are very low (<0.1 ng/mL).

PET imaging with FDG is not used for prostate cancer screening or detection, primary because prostate cancer does not routinely exhibit a glycolytic phenotype. In addition, small malignant lesions may be below detection limits of PET.[4] Moreover, tracer excretion through the kidney into the bladder obscures the inspection of the prostate bed on FDG-PET images (which could be remedied partly with the use of PET/CT imaging).

Tumor recurrence is most frequently established because of rising serum PSA levels. If tumor recurrence is confined to the prostate bed, localized salvage therapy can be curative. However, if rising PSA levels originate from distant disease, local salvage therapy is no longer an option because it is associated with considerable morbidity without improving survival.

The long-term outcome of patients who have biochemical disease recurrence after either prostatectomy or radiation therapy is correlated with pre–salvage therapy serum PSA levels.[5,6] Therefore, the site of recurrence must be detected as early as possible during relapse. Unfortunately, rising serum PSA levels, the rate of PSA rise (PSA velocity), the interval to PSA relapse, and pathologic features of the primary tumor do not accurately discriminate between local and distant disease.[7,8]

METASTATIC DISEASE

Advances in diagnostic imaging may result in better selection of patients for adjuvant local

The authors declare no conflicts of interest. The authors have nothing to disclose.
Department of Molecular and Medical Pharmacology, Division of Ahmanson Biological Imaging, David Geffen School of Medicine, Nuclear Medicine, CHS-AR 243, University of California Los Angeles, 10833 Le Conte Avenue, Los Angeles, CA 90095, USA
* Corresponding author.
E-mail address: jczernin@mednet.ucla.edu (J. Czernin).

PET Clin 4 (2009) 163–172
doi:10.1016/j.cpet.2009.05.001

versus systemic therapy. The usefulness of CT or MR imaging was recently investigated prospectively in 375 patients who were at intermediate or high risk for lymph node metastases.[9] For MR imaging, a novel lymph node–specific contrast agent (ferumoxtran-10, consisting of ultrasmall particles of iron oxide) was used. These particles migrate from the vascular space into the interstitial space, are taken up by macrophages, and are then cleared through lymphatic vessels to finally accumulate in lymph nodes. Because of hemodynamic alterations in the regional lymphatic system induced by metastatic lesions, fewer particle-containing macrophages arrive in lymph nodes harboring metastatic disease, resulting in different signal intensities on MR images.

Using histology as the gold standard, the specificity of MR and CT imaging was high at greater than 90%. However, MR imaging was significantly more sensitive than CT (82% versus 34%; $P<.05$). Thus, MR imaging might play an increasing role in detecting lymph node metastases in patients who have evidence of biochemical recurrence.

Although MR imaging is frequently used for initial staging of local lymph node involvement, bone involvement is detected using bone scans in patients who have PSA levels of greater than 10 ng/mL. Extensive CT or MR imaging surveys for distant disease are limited to patients in whom metastatic disease is highly suspected.

FDG-PET has also been used for detecting metastatic prostate cancer and has a considerable impact on patient management.[10–12]

Seltzer and colleagues[13] showed that antibody imaging targeting prostate-specific membrane antigen ([111]-indium Prostascint) has limited usefulness for detecting metastatic prostate cancer. This imaging probe detected distant disease in only 1 of 6 patients who had known metastases.

Metastatic disease can also be detected with conventional bone scans, ^{18}F-sodium fluoride PET/(CT) bone scans, MR imaging, or CT imaging. None of these techniques alone is well suited for monitoring therapeutic responses.[14]

Current therapeutic options in advanced disease are limited and mainly include hormonal treatments. However, several targeted therapeutic approaches are under investigation but have not yet reached clinical routine.[15] Imaging is unlikely to play a role in detecting primary prostate cancer. However, imaging approaches would be useful that would (1) allow for detection of and discrimination between local recurrence and distant metastatic disease, and (2) permit the monitoring of tumor responses to novel therapeutic approaches. Molecular PET imaging probes that have been investigated for these indications include [11]C- or

[18]F-choline, ^{18}F-labeled amino acids, and antibody approaches.[16]

This article focuses on the potential ability of ^{11}C-acetate to improve care of patients who have prostate cancer. The article first discusses the biochemical processes targeted by ^{11}C-acetate imaging, explores its biodistribution and dosimetry, and then reviews the limited data on imaging primary, recurrent, and metastatic disease with this metabolic imaging probe.

BIOLOGIC CORRELATES OF ^{11}C-ACETATE UPTAKE IN PROSTATE CANCER

Major metabolic pathways for acetate include the tricarboxylic acid (TCA) cycle,[17] and lipid and cholesterol synthesis.

[11]C-acetate is actively transported across cell membranes through monocarboxylate transporters.[18] After conversion to acetyl-CoA in the mitochondria, the metabolic fate of ^{11}C-acetate is diverse. In tissues with high rates of oxidative metabolism, acetyl-CoA enters the TCA cycle, resulting in carbon dioxide production.

[11]C-acetate was initially used to measure myocardial oxidative metabolism with external gamma probes[19] or PET.[20,21] In both approaches, the myocardial tracer extraction and clearance kinetics were studied under various conditions (eg, control, ischemia, reperfusion, increased oxygen demand) and ^{11}C-acetate clearance was correlated closely with myocardial oxygen consumption. [11]C clearance measured externally with PET corresponded to carbon dioxide production and thus TCA cycle activity.

However, increased oxidative metabolism is highly unlikely to account for tumor retention of ^{11}C-acetate. Its retention in prostate cancer is most likely caused by increased fatty acid synthesis (**Fig. 1**). Fatty acid synthase (FAS) plays important roles in the de novo synthesis of fatty acids from acetyl-CoA, malonyl-CoA, and NADPH in normal and abnormal tissues.[22] Its normal biologic functions include the production of lecithin for surfactant, supply of fatty components of breast milk, and conversion and storage of energy in liver and adipose tissue. Human cancer cells do not store lipids but rather incorporate them into membranes as phospholipids.

FAS is overexpressed in many human cancers, particularly prostate cancer.[23] The degree of its overexpression seems to correlate with tumor aggressiveness[24] and is linked to various oncogenic signal transduction pathways.[2] FAS affects the phospholipid content of membrane fractions and helps control the lipid composition of membrane microdomains, which might affect

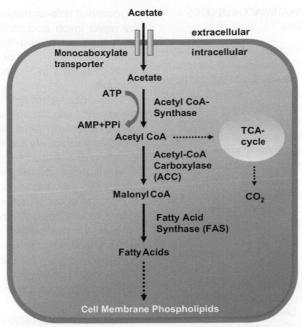

Fig. 1. Simplified schematic of fatty acid synthesis: fatty acid synthase catalyzes the de-novo synthesis of fatty acid from acetyl-CoA, malonyl-CoA, and NADPH. After several reactions and modifications, fatty acids are incorporated into membranes as phospholipids. CO_2, carbon dioxide; PPi, pyrophosphate; TCA, tricarboxylic acid.

signal transduction, cell migration, and other processes.[25]

Blocking fatty acid synthase with small interfering RNA or a small molecule inhibitor causes tumor cell death through the caspase 8–mediated apoptotic pathway.[17] It also decreases ^{11}C-acetate uptake in various prostate cancer cell lines.[25] Brusselmans and colleagues[26] provided additional evidence for the critical role of lipid synthesis in maintaining tumor cell proliferation and viability in prostate cancer. They used RNA interference to silence acetyl-CoA-carboxylase in malignant LNCaP prostate cancer cell lines, resulting in growth arrest and apoptosis. Acetyl-CoA-carboxylase is the rate-limiting enzyme in the fatty acid synthesis pathway that produces malonyl-CoA. Blocking this enzyme reduces cellular ^{11}C-acetate uptake even more potently than inhibiting FAS (by >80%).[27]

Malonyl-CoA is a substrate for fatty acid synthesis and is a negative regulator of fatty acid oxidation. Inhibiting this enzyme with soraphen A, a macrocyclic polyketide, reduced the phospholipid content of prostate cancer cells and caused growth arrest of various prostate cancer cell lines in the G0–G1 cell cycle phase.[28] Inhibiting this enzyme also resulted in a switch to fatty acid oxidation.

The tumor microenvironment also seems to be a significant determinant of the tumor uptake of

[11]C-acetate, at least in cell culture. Hara and colleagues[29] provided insights into the relationship between glucose and fatty acid metabolism in human prostate cancer cell lines under normoxic and hypoxic conditions. They examined the uptake of tritiated choline, ^{14}C-acetate, and ^{18}F-FDG under normoxic and anoxic conditions in one androgen-independent and another androgen-dependent prostate cancer cell line. FDG uptake was highest after 4 hours of anoxia. Under anoxic conditions, ^{11}C-acetate uptake was also increased in androgen-dependent, but not -independent, cell lines, whereas choline uptake was reduced in all cell lines. Under aerobic conditions, uptake of choline was higher than that of ^{14}C-acetate, which was still more than five times higher than that of FDG. Androgen depletion resulted in low uptake of all three tracers.

This study confirms several clinical observations: (1) FDG imaging might be useful in patients who have advanced prostate cancer whose metastatic lesions are likely to be hypoxic and hence exhibit a glycolytic phenotype; (2) ^{11}C-acetate or ^{11}C/^{18}F-choline imaging might be useful for detecting early, "well-oxygenated" disease; and (3) all three probes might be limited in their sensitivity for detecting prostate cancer tissue in patients undergoing antiandrogen treatments. Hara and colleagues[29] discuss the biochemical alterations underlying these phenotypic changes.

BIODISTRIBUTION AND PHARMACOKINETICS OF ^{11}C-ACETATE IN HUMANS

In control rodents, the pancreas exhibits the highest ^{11}C-acetate uptake 20 minutes after injection. Within 1 hour, activity clears from all organs, except the pancreas. Tumor ^{11}C-acetate uptake was clearly visible at 30 minutes.[30]

Time activity curves obtained from regions of interest placed over serially acquired PET images obtained in a healthy volunteer are shown in **Fig. 2**.[31] Early tracer uptake in tissues such as salivary glands, myocardium, and kidneys is followed by rapid clearance. As in rodents and baboons,[30] early tracer accumulation is also noted in the pancreas. **Fig. 3** shows the normal biodistribution of ^{11}C-acetate in a healthy subject.

At later time points, some bowel activity is noted. The whole body biodistribution of ^{11}C-acetate differs from that of FDG in that its accumulation in the urinary bladder is minimal (see **Fig. 3**). Therefore, the prostate bed can be readily inspected on whole-body ^{11}C-acetate images.

Tracer kinetics in tumors differ from that in normal tissues, such as the myocardium. In tumors, a plateau phase follows flow-dependent tracer delivery that is consistent with ^{11}C-acetate retention in tumor cells (**Fig. 4**).[32] In contrast, myocardial time–activity curves are characterized by rapid tracer accumulation representing blood flow that is followed by rapid tracer clearance when acetate is metabolized in the TCA cycle. More than 80% of ^{11}C-acetate is cleared after 20 minutes.

These discrepant time–activity curves between tumor and heart strongly suggest that the retention of ^{11}C-acetate in tumor tissue is largely unrelated to TCA cycle activity and is accounted for by incorporation of acetate into the lipid pool.

In summary, the degree to which various lipid metabolic pathways and their individual steps contribute to the retention of ^{11}C-acetate in prostate cancer tissue are incompletely understood. However, incorporation into the lipid pool, and more specifically into membrane lipids,[33] seems to largely account for the preferential retention of ^{11}C-acetate in prostate cancer, whereas fatty acid oxidation plays a only a limited role, if any.

CLINICAL STUDIES USING ^{11}C-ACETATE

[11]C-Acetate Dosimetry

Organ dosimetry was established[31] from studies in 6 healthy volunteers who underwent serial whole-body PET imaging after the intravenous injection of 525 MBq (14.2 mCi) of ^{11}C acetate. The organs

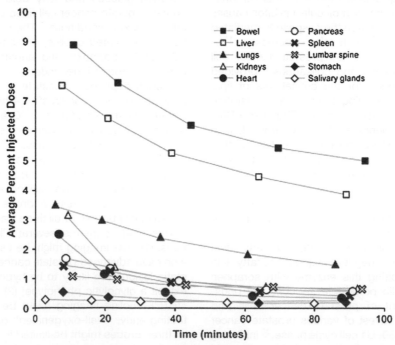

Fig. 2. Tissue time–activity curves from serial ^{11}C-acetate images obtained in healthy subjects. Note that activity in pancreas and liver remains high at 100 minutes after tracer injection. (*From* Seltzer M, Jahan S, Sparks R, et al. Radiation dose estimates in humans for ^{11}C-acetate whole-body PET. J Nucl Med 2004;45:1233–6; with permission.)

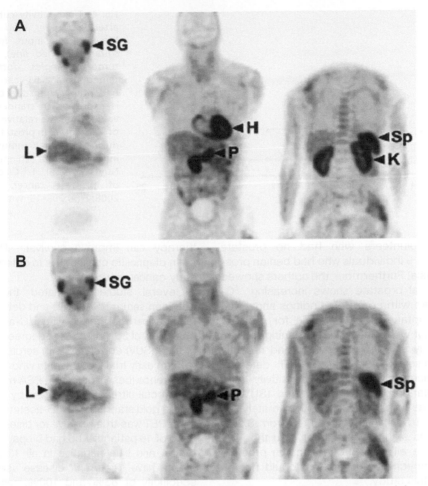

Fig. 3. Normal biodistribution of ¹¹C-acetate in a healthy subject. Images in the upper row (*A*) were obtained 2 minutes after tracer injection, and those at the bottom (*B*) were acquired 28 minutes after injection of ¹¹C-acetate. H, heart; K, kidneys; L, liver; P, pancreas; SG, salivary glands; Sp, spleen. (*From* Seltzer M, Jahan S, Sparks R, et al. Radiation dose estimates in humans for ¹¹C-acetate whole-body PET. J Nucl Med 2004;45:1233–6; with permission.)

receiving the highest doses were the pancreas (critical organ receiving 0.017 mGy/MBq), bowel, kidneys, and spleen.

Clinical Imaging Protocols

Because of the short half-life of ¹¹C-acetate, imaging commences from 2 to 10 minutes after tracer injection. Injected doses range from 555 to 1110 MBq (15–30 mCi). In patients who have suspected recurrence, images of the pelvis are acquired first. Imaging times per bed position range from 5 to 10 minutes to achieve adequate activity count rates. Depending on the clinical question to be addressed, the imaging field is subsequently expanded to include the abdomen and, if needed, the chest.

When PET/CT is used, a CT scan with or without intravenous contrast is acquired first. This is used both for attenuation correction and as a diagnostic CT study. The extent of the imaging field depends on the clinical question asked, patient stage, and individual patient risk profile for distant metastatic disease.

Detection of Prostate Cancer

One of the first questions to be addressed in clinical studies is whether the degree of ¹¹C-acetate permits to differentiate normal prostate tissue from benign hyperplasia and prostate cancer. Using a conventional PET scanner, Kato and colleagues[34] demonstrated in 36 research volunteers that the degree of ¹¹C-acetate uptake was comparable among 6 patients who had prostate

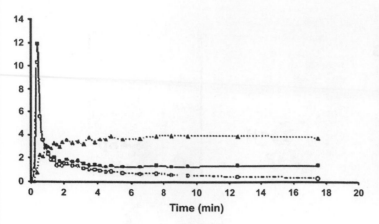

Fig. 4. Time–activity curves from iliac arteries (*squares, solid line*), metabolite-corrected input function (*open squares, dashed line*), and prostate tumor (*triangles, dotted line*) obtained from a 65-year-old man who had primary prostate cancer. Uptake is expressed in standardized uptake value. Note the relative stable activity of ^{11}C-acetate in prostate cancer tissue during the first 20 minutes after tracer injection. (*From* Schiepers C, Hoh CK, Nuyts J, et al. 1-^{11}C-acetate kinetics of prostate cancer. J Nucl Med 2008;49(2):206–15; with permission.)

cancer, 21 volunteers who had no prostate pathology, and 9 individuals who had benign prostate hyperplasia. Furthermore, the authors showed that the normal prostate shows increasing ^{11}C-acetate uptake with age. Both findings show that ^{11}C-acetate uptake is not specific for prostate cancer and not well suited as a screening tool.

In one study of 22 patients who had recently diagnosed disease, ^{11}C-acetate PET detected prostate cancer with a higher sensitivity than FDG. The standardized uptake value (SUV) of ^{11}C-acetate as measured at approximately 20 minutes after tracer injection ranged from 3.2 to 9.9 (which was significantly higher than the FDG SUV). Because all patients had known prostate cancer, the specificity of the test could not be examined in this study.

In summary, the available literature on primary prostate cancer detection with ^{11}C-acetate is limited. However, it suggests that ^{11}C-acetate cannot be proposed for prostate cancer screening (because of the comparable tracer uptake levels among cancer, hyperplasia, and even normal prostate tissue). Nevertheless, the data show that ^{11}C-acetate uptake is visible and measurable through SUV in prostate tissue. This finding is important because the most interesting potential application of ^{11}C-acetate imaging is for detecting prostate cancer recurrence. For this indication, the issue of specificity is clinically much less relevant.

Recurrent and Metastatic Prostate Cancer

Biochemical evidence of prostate cancer recurrence after radical prostatectomy or radiation treatment, frequently defined as a serum PSA level of 0.2 ng/mL, precedes the clinical manifestations of recurrent disease. Once metastatic disease develops, the prognosis is poor, with an overall patient survival of 5 years.[35] In patients who have locally recurrent disease, salvage radiation

therapy can improve survival.[6] Therefore, the main diagnostic challenge is to detect and localize early cancer recurrence.

Several studies evaluated the relationship between serum PSA levels and detection of prostate cancer recurrence with ^{11}C-acetate PET. In one study of 25 patients, the degree of ^{11}C-acetate uptake (SUV) correlated with serum PSA levels.[36]

In an early trial[37] of patients who had suspected recurrence (based on serum PSA measurements), transrectal ultrasound followed by biopsy served as the gold standard for ^{11}C-acetate imaging findings. PET was true positive for disease recurrence in 15 of 18 patients who had biopsy-proven recurrence, and true negative in all 13 patients who didn't have recurrent disease (sensitivity and specificity of 83% and 100%, respectively). In this study, PET was positive in 4 of 5 patients who had biopsy-proven cancers and serum PSA levels of less than 2 ng/mL.

A reasonable detectability of disease in patients who had low PSA levels was also recently reported by Albrecht and colleagues.[38] In their study, 17 patients were imaged after primary radiation therapy and 15 after radical surgery. All had biochemical evidence of recurrent disease. PSA levels were significantly higher after radiation treatment (6 ng/mL) than after radical prostatectomy (0.4 ng/mL). PET and non–contrast-enhanced CT images were fused using a commercially available fusion software. An arbitrary SUV threshold of 2.0 was selected for discriminating between equivocal and positive PET results.

In the 17 patients who had undergone radiation therapy, PET suggested local recurrences in 14 and was true positive in 5 of 6 who had positive biopsy results. The detection of bone metastases with ^{11}C-acetate was, however, limited when bone scans and CT were used as reference standards. ^{11}C-acetate suggested recurrence in 9 of 15 patients who underwent primary surgery and

PET was similarly sensitive (approximately 60%) in patients who had serum PSA levels of less than 0.8 ng/mL.

In contrast, poor detection of recurrent disease in patients who had low serum PSA levels was reported by the St. Louis group, who used ¹¹C-acetate and ¹⁸F-FDG PET imaging in 46 patients.[39] Their study group included patients who had undergone radiation and others who underwent surgery as primary treatment. Various clinical studies, including bone scans, CT scans, and biopsy, served as reference standards for the PET findings.

As a physiologic variant, the authors noted frequent mild ¹¹C-acetate in inguinal lymph nodes (not reported elsewhere) and considered this a normal pattern. ¹¹C-acetate images suggested with intermediate or high probability the presence of disease in 59% of the patients, whereas FDG-PET imaging suggested disease in only 17% of the participants. Notably, ¹¹C acetate PET was positive in 59% of patients who had PSA levels of greater than 3 ng/mL but only in 4% of those who had levels less than 3 ng/mL.

Based on extensive clinical experience, Reske and colleagues[40] suggested that PET/CT imaging or fused PET and MR images allow for better detection of local recurrence. This notion is supported by the results of a small pilot trial that used ¹¹C-acetate PET/CT in 11 patients who had serum PSA levels of less than 0.3 ng/mL. The authors identified the site of recurrence in 6 of 11 patients.[41]

However, even with PET/CT, the site of recurrence might be difficult to identify in patients who have low serum PSA levels. In one study, software fusion of CT or MR and PET images in 50 patients who had biochemical evidence for recurrent disease[42] resulted in markedly improved accuracy in disease detection and localization. Image fusion changed interpretation from equivocal to normal in 10% and from equivocal to abnormal in 18% of the lesions. Management was affected in 28% of the patients. A gold standard (biopsy) for verification of PET findings was only available in a small subset of patients. In general, patients who had false-negative PET findings had low serum PSA values (median 0.9 ng/mL). However, the authors correctly noted that in four of the six patients who had a PSA ranging from to 2.6 to 13 ng/mL after radical prostatectomy, the ¹¹C-acetate scan was also false-negative.

Using ¹¹C-acetate PET/(CT), Sandblom and colleagues[43] enrolled 20 patients who had elevated PSA levels that ranged from 0.5 to 8.1 ng/mL after radical prostatectomy. All underwent ¹¹C-acetate PET/CT imaging (**Fig. 5**) in addition

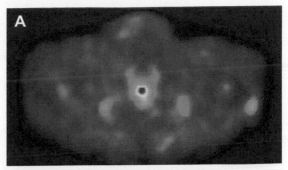

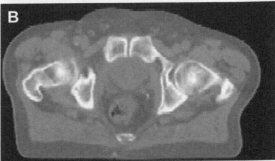

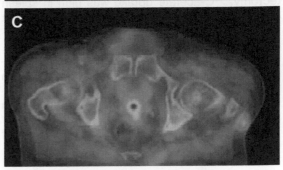

Fig. 5. ¹¹C-acetate positron emission tomography (PET) (A), non–contrast-enhanced computed tomography (CT) (B), and fused PET/CT images (C) in a patient who had biochemical recurrence and a serum prostate-specific antigen level of 2.5 ng/mL. The lesion in the prostate bed had a maximum standardized uptake value of 5. Note the absence of tracer accumulation in the urinary bladder. (*From* Sandblom G, Sörensen J, Lundin N, et al. Positron emission tomography with C11-acetate for tumor detection and localization in patients with prostate-specific antigen relapse after radical prostatectomy. Urology 2006;67(5):996–1000; with permission.)

to all standard examinations performed for identifying cancer recurrence sites. ¹¹C-acetate identified disease sites in 75% of patients. All patients who had positive PET scans had serum PSA levels greater than 2.0 ng/mL, and their SUVs ranged from 2.0 to 8.1. False-positive findings occurred in three patients. One exhibited tracer uptake in the chest, which was subsequently confirmed to represent non–small cell lung cancer, whereas two other patients had inflammatory changes, one in the esophagus and the other one in the mediastinum. These findings confirm that ^{11}C-acetate uptake is not cancer-specific but rather a probe of lipid metabolism that can also be altered in inflammatory disease.

In summary, recurrent prostate cancer can be detected with ^{11}C-acetate, but because detectability seems to be correlated with serum PSA levels, detectability is limited in patients who have serum PSA levels less than 3 ng/mL.

COMPARATIVE STUDIES

Several groups compared the diagnostic performance of ^{11}C-acetate and other metabolic PET imaging probes in patients who had prostate cancer. A small pilot trial of 12 patients who had prostate cancer[44] compared the biodistribution of ^{11}C-acetate and ^{11}C-choline (a substrate of choline kinase that is also incorporated into membrane lipids) in patients after initial diagnosis, at biochemical recurrence, or after radical prostatectomy. ^{11}C-acetate uptake was high in spleen and pancreas, with ^{11}C-choline uptake most prominent in liver and kidneys. Importantly, ^{11}C-acetate was not excreted into the bladder, whereas urinary excretion was variable for ^{11}C-choline. In terms of tumor uptake, however, both imaging probes missed detection of small prostatic lesions and 3 of 13 small metastatic lymph nodes that were confirmed using surgery/pathology. Thus, the diagnostic performance of both imaging probes was comparable.

In another study, Vees and colleagues[41] compared these probes in 20 patients, imaging 10 with ^{11}C-choline and the remaining 10 with ^{11}C-acetate. Both tracers provided a comparable cancer detection rate, with abnormal local tracer uptake in 5 of 10 patients imaged with ^{11}C-choline and 6 of 10 imaged with ^{11}C-acetate. The authors concluded that both tracers detect approximately 50% of cancer recurrences, but that endorectal MR imaging, which detected 15 of 18 recurrences, was superior.

Fricke and colleagues[36] compared lesion detectability using ^{18}F-FDG and ^{11}C-acetate imaging in a small, heterogeneous population of patients who had prostate cancer, including those who had primary cancer, those who had suspected relapse, and some who had metastatic disease. Overall sensitivity of the acetate approach was 83%, which was slightly better than that for FDG (75%). Local recurrence was better detected with[11]C-acetate, whereas distant disease was better visualized with ^{18}F-FDG.

Taken together, those studies suggest that [11]C-/^{18}F-choline and ^{11}C-acetate seem to have a comparable accuracy for detecting local recurrence, whereas FDG-PET might be better suited for detecting metastatic disease.

[18]F-Fluoroacetate

Because of its short half-life of 20.4 minutes, the use of ^{11}C-labeled PET imaging probes requires an on-site cyclotron. With this limitation in mind, the Washington University group synthesized ^{18}F-fluoroacetate and studied its biodistribution in mice and baboons using a small animal PET system and human scanner.[30] Although defluorination occurred in rodents, it was not observed in baboons. However, the biodistribution of [11]C- and ^{18}F-acetate differed. For instance, ^{11}C-acetate blood activity was lower than that of the fluorinated analog. However, tumor uptake of ^{18}F-acetate was five times higher that than of ^{11}C-acetate 30 minutes after intravenous injection. ^{18}F-fluoroacetate tumor-to-background ratios (other than blood) from various tissues were consistently higher than those for ^{11}C-acetate. Thus, this probe shows promise for imaging prostate and other cancers that exhibit low FDG uptake.

SUMMARY

[11]C-acetate can be used to image prostate cancer, particularly recurrent disease. Limitations include its low sensitivity for disease detection at low serum PSA levels. The routine use of PET/CT imaging will further improve the diagnostic accuracy of this approach.

Importantly, novel therapeutic approaches targeting tumor lipid metabolism are under development.[45] Imaging of tumor lipid metabolism with [11]C-/^{18}F-acetate may provide a valuable readout for assessing drug effects on the lipogenic phenotype in vivo.

REFERENCES

1. Warburg O, Posener K, Negelein E VIII. The metabolism of cancer cells. Biochem Zeitschr 1924;152:129–69.
2. Plathow C, Weber W. Tumor cell metabolism imaging. J Nucl Med 2008;49(Suppl 2):43S–63S.
3. Crupp M, Oesterling J. Prostate-specific antigen, digital rectal examination, and transrectal ultrasonography: their roles in diagnosing early prostate cancer. Mayo Clin Proc 1993;68:297–306.
4. Hofer C, Laubenbacher C, Block T, et al. Fluorine-18-fluorodeoxyglucose positron emission tomography is useless for the detection of local recurrence after radical prostatectomy. Eur Urol 1999;36:31–5.

5. Cox J, Gallagher M, Hammond E, et al. Consensus statements on radiation therapy of prostate cancer: guidelines for prostate re-biopsy after radiation and for radiation therapy with rising prostate-specific antigen levels after radical prostatectomy. American Society for Therapeutic Radiology and Oncology Consensus Panel. J Clin Oncol 1999;17:1155–63.

6. Stephenson AJ, Shariat SF, Zelefsky MJ, et al. Salvage radiotherapy for recurrent prostate cancer after radical prostatectomy. JAMA 2004;291(11):1325–32.

7. Leibman B, Dilioglugil O, Wheeler T, et al. Distant metastasis after radical prostatectomy in patients without an elevated serum prostate specific antigen level. Cancer 1995;76:2530–4.

8. Partin A, Oesterling J. The clinical usefulness of prostate specific antigen: update 1994. J Urol 1994;152:1358–68.

9. Heesakkers RA, Hövels AM, Jager GJ, et al. MRI with a lymph-node-specific contrast agent as an alternative to CT scan and lymph-node dissection in patients with prostate cancer: a prospective multi-cohort study. Lancet Oncol 2008;9(9):850–6.

10. Hillner B, Siegel B, Shields A, et al. The impact of positron emission tomography (PET) on expected management during cancer treatment: findings of the National Oncologic PET Registry. Cancer 2009; 115:410–8.

11. Hillner BE, Liu D, Coleman RE, et al. The national oncologic PET registry (NOPR): design and analysis plan. J Nucl Med 2007;48(11):1901–8.

12. Hillner BE, Siegel BA, Liu D, et al. Impact of positron emission tomography/computed tomography and positron emission tomography (PET) alone on expected management of patients with cancer: initial results from the National Oncologic PET Registry. J Clin Oncol 2008;26(13):2155–61.

13. Seltzer M, Barbaric Z, Belldegrun A, et al. Comparison of helical computerized tomography, positron emission tomography and monoclonal antibody scans for evaluation of lymph node metastases in patients with prostate specific antigen relapse after treatment for localized prostate cancer. J Urol 1999;162:1322–8.

14. Israel O, Goldberg A, Nachtigal A, et al. FDG-PET and CT patterns of bone metastases and their relationship to previously administered anti-cancer therapy. Eur J Nucl Med Mol Imaging 2006;33(11):1280–4.

15. Chen Y, Sawyers C, Scher H. Targeting the androgen receptor pathway in prostate cancer. Curr Opin Pharmacol 2008;8(4):440–8.

16. Larson S, Schöder H. Advances in positron emission tomography applications for urologic cancers. Curr Opin Urol 2008;18:65–70.

17. Knowles LM, Yang C, Osterman A, et al. Inhibition of fatty-acid synthase induces caspase-8-mediated tumor cell apoptosis by up-regulating DDIT4. J Biol Chem 2008;283(46):31378–84.

18. Waniewski RA, Martin DL. Preferential utilization of acetate by astrocytes is attributable to transport. J Neurosci 1998;18(14):5225–33.

19. Brown M, Marshall DR, Sobel BE, et al. Delineation of myocardial oxygen utilization with carbon-11-labeled acetate. Circulation 1987;76(3):687–96.

20. Buxton D, Nienaber C, Luxen A, et al. Noninvasive quantitation of regional myocardial oxygen consumption in vivo with [1-^{11}C]acetate and dynamic positron emission tomography. Circulation 1989;79:134–42.

21. Buxton DB, Schwaiger M, Nguyen A, et al. Radio-labeled acetate as a tracer of myocardial tricarboxylic acid cycle flux. Circ Res 1988;63(3): 628–34.

22. Kuhajda FP. Fatty acid synthase and cancer: new application of an old pathway. Cancer Res 2006; 66:5977–80.

23. Baron A, Migita T, Tang D, et al. Fatty acid synthase: a metabolic oncogene in prostate cancer? J Cell Biochem 2003;91:47–53.

24. Epstein J, Carmichael M, Partin A. OA-519 (fatty acid synthase) as an independent predictor of pathologic state in adenocarcinoma of the prostate. Urology 1995;45:81–6.

25. Swinnen J, Van Veldhoven P, Timmermans L, et al. Fatty acid synthase drives the synthesis of phospho-lipids partitioning into detergent-resistant membrane microdomains. Biochem Biophys Res Commun 2003;302(4):898–903.

26. Brusselmans K, De Schrijver E, Verhoeven G, et al. RNA interference-mediated silencing of the acetyl-CoA-carboxylase-alpha gene induces growth inhibition and apoptosis of prostate cancer cells. Cancer Res 2005;65:6719–25.

27. Vavere A, Kridel S, Wheeler F, et al. 1-^{11}C-acetate as a PET radiopharmaceutical for imaging fatty acid synthase expression in prostate cancer. J Nucl Med 2008;49:327–34.

28. Beckers A, Organe S, Timmermans L, et al. Chemical inhibition of acetyl-CoA carboxylase induces growth arrest and cytotoxicity selectively in cancer cells. Cancer Res 2007;67:8180–7.

29. Hara T, Bansal A, DeGrado T. Effect of hypoxia on the uptake of [methyl-^{3}H]choline, [1-^{14}C] acetate and [^{18}F]FDG in cultured prostate cancer cells. Nucl Med Biol 2006;33(8):977–84.

30. Ponde D, Dence C, Oyama N, et al. ^{18}F-fluoroace-tate: a potential acetate analog for prostate tumor imaging—in vivo evaluation of ^{18}F-fluoroacetate versus ^{11}C-acetate. J Nucl Med 2007;48:420–8.

31. Seltzer M, Jahan S, Sparks R, et al. Radiation dose estimates in humans for ^{11}C-acetate whole-body PET. J Nucl Med 2004;45:1233–6.

32. Schiepers C, Hoh CK, Nuyts J, et al. 1-^{11}C-acetate kinetics of prostate cancer. J Nucl Med 2008;49(2): 206–15.

33. Yoshimoto M, Waki A, Yonekura Y, et al. Characterization of acetate metabolism in tumor cells in relation to cell proliferation: acetate metabolism in tumor cells. Nucl Med Biol 2001;28(2):117–22.

34. Kato T, Tsukamoto E, Kuge Y, et al. Accumulation of [11C]acetate in normal prostate and benign prostatic hyperplasia: comparison with prostate cancer. Eur J Nucl Med Mol Imaging 2002; 29(11):1492–5.

35. Pound C, Partin A, Eisenberger M, et al. Natural history of progression after PSA elevation following radical prostatectomy. JAMA 1999;281:1591–7.

36. Fricke E, Machtens S, Hofmann M, et al. Positron emission tomography with 11C-acetate and 18F-FDG in prostate cancer patients. Eur J Nucl Med Mol Imaging 2003;30(4):607–11.

37. Kotzerke J, Volkmer B, Neumaier B, et al. Carbon-11 acetate positron emission tomography can detect local recurrence of prostate cancer. Eur J Nucl Med Mol Imaging 2002;29(10):1380–4.

38. Albrecht S, Buchegger F, Soloviev D, et al. 11C-acetate PET in the early evaluation of prostate cancer recurrence. Eur J Nucl Med Mol Imaging 2007;34(2):185–96.

39. Oyama N, Miller T, Dehdashti F, et al. 11C-acetate PET imaging of prostate cancer: detection of recurrent disease at PSA relapse. J Nucl Med 2003;44: 549–55.

40. Reske S, Blumstein N, Glatting G. PET und PET/CT in der Rezidivdiagnostik des Prostatakarzinoms [PET and PET/CT in relapsing prostate carcinoma]. Urologe A 2006;45(10):1240–50 [in German].

41. Vees H, Buchegger F, Albrecht S, et al. 18F-choline and/or 11C-acetate positron emission tomography: detection of residual or progressive subclinical disease at very low prostate-specific antigen values (<1 ng/mL) after radical prostatectomy. BJU Int 2007;99:1415–20.

42. Wachter S, Sandra T, Kurtaran A, et al. 11C-acetate positron emission tomography imaging and image fusion with computed tomography and magnetic resonance imaging in patients with recurrent prostate cancer. J Clin Oncol 2006;24:2513–9.

43. Sandblom G, Sörensen J, Lundin N, et al. Positron emission tomography with C11-acetate for tumor detection and localization in patients with prostate-specific antigen relapse after radical prostatectomy. Urology 2006;67(5):996–1000.

44. Kotzerke J, Volkmer B, Glatting G, et al. Intraindividual comparison of [11C]acetate and [11C]choline PET for detection of metastases of prostate cancer. Nuklearmedizin 2003;42:25–30.

45. Zhou W, Han W, Landree L. Fatty acid synthase inhibition activates AMP-activated protein kinase in SKOV3 human ovarian cancer cells. Cancer Res 2007;67:2964–71.

PET Imaging of Prostate Cancer Using Radiolabeled Choline

Mohsen Beheshti, MD, FEBNM, FASNC*,
Werner Langsteger, MD, FACE

KEYWORDS

• PET imaging • Radiolabeled choline • Prostate cancer

PET using 18F-fluorodeoxyglucose (FDG) has proved to be a promising modality for metabolic imaging of different tumors; however, the results in prostate cancer have been somewhat inconsistent.[1–7] Low FDG avidity of most prostate cancer cells and urinary activity are suggested as the main limitations of FDG PET for the evaluation of prostate cancer.[1]

Prostate cancer exhibits increased choline metabolism, which is the rationale for using radiolabeled choline for PET. The value of PET using 11C-choline and 18F-choline for the assessment of prostate cancer patients is discussed controversially, from encouraging results to limited usefulness.[8–13]

In this article, the authors describe the basic concepts of radiolabeled choline regarding pharmacokinetics, radiation dosimetry, synthesis, and biodistribution, in addition to advances concerning clinical PET using 11C- and 18F-choline in primary staging and restaging of prostate cancer patients.

PHARMACOKINETICS AND RADIATION DOSIMETRY

Choline is a quaternary ammonium base that is used as a precursor for the biosynthesis of phospholipids (eg, phosphatidylcholine [lecithin]), which are essential components of all cell membranes.[14,15] The first step in the synthesis of phosphatidylcholine is phosphorylation of choline, which is catalyzed by choline kinase (**Fig. 1**). Choline kinase is widely distributed in tissues such as brain, liver, and lung.[16] In the next step, phosphorylcholine is converted to cytidine diphosphate–choline and catalyzed by cytidine triphosphate by means of phosphocholine cytydyltransferase.[17]

In addition, choline participates in two other enzyme-catalyzed pathways: oxidation and acetylation (see **Fig. 1**).[15] Following the oxidation pathway, choline is oxidized to betaine aldehyde, which is then converted into betaine by choline oxidase, particularly in the liver and kidney. Betaine serves as an organic osmolyte in the cell to maintain cell volume homeostasis.[18]

Only a small amount of choline is acetylated with acetyl coenzyme A to acetylcholine and catalyzed by choline acetyltransferase, which is highly concentrated in the cholinergic nerve terminals. This pathway is important because acetylcholine is a neurotransmitter.[19]

Carcinogenesis is characterized by increased cell proliferation. It has been suggested that malignant transformation of cells is associated with the enhancement of choline kinase activity, resulting in increased levels of phosphorylcholine.[14] Furthermore, it is shown that progressive tumors contain large amounts of phospholipids, mainly phosphatidylcholine.[20] It has been shown that phospholipids (eg, phosphatidylcholine) may also induce signaling processes within cells and consequently influence cell proliferation and differentiation.[21]

Many phosphorus 31 magnetic resonance spectroscopy studies have shown a high content of phosphorylcholine in most cancers, whereas in corresponding normal tissues, this choline metabolite is present at low levels,[22–24] providing

Department of Nuclear Medicine & Endocrinology, PET-CT Center Linz, St. Vincent's Hospital, Seilerstaette 4, A–4020 Linz, Austria
* Corresponding author.
E-mail address: mohsen.beheshti@bhs.at (M. Beheshti).

PET Clin 4 (2009) 173–184
doi:10.1016/j.cpet.2009.06.003

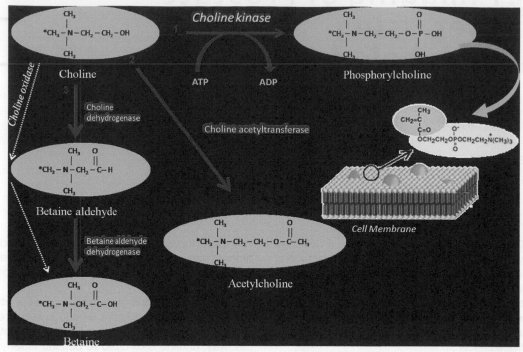

Fig. 1. Schematic presentation of the three main metabolic pathways of radiolabeled choline: 1 = phosphorylation; 2 = acetylation; 3 = oxidation. Labeling positions are indicated by an asterisk.

the rationale for the use of radiolabeled choline in oncologic PET studies.

Roivainen and colleagues[15] demonstrated the biodistribution and metabolism of 11C-choline in rats and humans. They showed that after an initial rapid metabolism, the ratio of 11C-choline to 11C-betaine (the major metabolites in human arterial blood plasma) remained constant after 20 minutes. These investigators attributed the late clearance pattern as reflecting the metabolism of 11C-choline and 11C-betaine and the subsequent clearance of the latter by the urinary system, because most 11C in arterial plasma is in the form of 11C-betaine after 5 minutes post tracer administration. Although most of the circulating 11C-choline in blood is transported to tissues, it did not disappear totally from blood during the PET study (ie, 40 minutes).

The practical advantages of working with the longer-lived radioisotope 18F ($T_{1/2}$ = 110 minutes) led Hara and colleagues[25] to synthesize and evaluate the choline analog 18F-fluoroethylcholine (FECH). In vitro experiments showed incorporation into tumor cells by active transport, intracellular phosphorylation, and a final integration into phospholipids.

DeGrado and colleagues[26] developed an "18F-fluoromethylated" choline derivative (hydrogen atom of choline substituted by 18F), anticipating

that this tracer would mimic choline transport and metabolism more closely than FECH because of its structural similarity, with lower excretion of 18F radioactivity. Also, increased uptake of fluoromethyl-dimethyl-2-hydroxyethylammonium (18F-fluorocholine; FCH) has been shown in PC-3 prostate cancer cells compared with FECH. Furthermore, these investigators measured the in vitro phosphorylation rates of FCH and FECH using yeast choline kinase and showed that the phosphorylation rate of FCH is comparable with that of choline, whereas the phosphorylation rate of FECH is 30% lower. Bender and colleagues[27] compared both derivatives and reported a 1.5 to 3.0 times higher uptake of FCH in known metastases and in normal organs (1.2–2.5 times higher) compared with FECH. In addition, both 18F-labeled choline derivatives showed a significant urinary excretion.

In another study, DeGrado and colleagues[28] showed the biodistribution of FCH in humans. The blood clearance for FCH was found to be very rapid, with nonappreciable change in the biodistribution pattern seen at more than 10 minutes post intravenous administration. When comparing these data with those of Roivainen and colleagues[15] obtained with 11C-choline, it is presumed that FCH may not undergo the oxidative pathway and therefore does not exhibit the later clearance pattern observed with 11C-choline. This insignificant tissue clearance with FCH administration may also reflect specific metabolic trapping of the tracer in the phosphorylation pathway and further incorporation of the radiolabel into phospholipids, as shown in cultured prostate cancer cells.[29] Further investigations have been suggested to confirm whether the presence of the fluorine atom of FCH renders the molecule less appropriate for oxidation and subsequent clearance than natural choline.[28]

The kidney is the dose-critical organ and limits administration levels of FCH to 4.07 MBq/kg, with an effective dose equivalent of 0.01 Sv for women and men.[28]

SYNTHESIS

In general, the production of all choline derivatives is based on the alkylation of dimethylaminoethanol (DMAE) on solid phase or in a reactor system. 11C-choline is synthesized by the 11C-methylation of DMAE on an 18C solid phase, and the final product is purified by a cation exchange cartridge followed by a formulation in saline.[30,31] In a similar way, Hara and colleagues[25] described the synthesis of FECH by the production of 18F-fluoroethyltosylate and the subsequent fluoroethylation of DMAE in a reaction vessel. The final product is purified by high-performance liquid chromatography (HPLC) separation.[32]

The synthesis of FCH starts with the synthesis of the 18F-fluoromethylation agent 18F-fluoromethylbromide by the reaction of 18F-fluoride with dibromomethane, followed by the conversion of the intermediate to the more reactive 18F-fluoromethyltriflate.[32,33] Then, DMAE is fluoromethylated on solid phase, and the final product is purified as described for 11C-choline. Meanwhile, the synthesis process could be fully automated and integrated in a sterile disposable kit system.[34] The quality-control of all choline derivatives is performed analogous. The radiochemical purity of 11C-choline, FECH, and FCH is determined by HPLC. A central point in the quality control of both tracers is the quantitation of DMAE, which is suggested to be performed by HPLC or by gas chromatography.[32]

BIODISTRIBUTION (11C-CHOLINE VERSUS 18F-CHOLINE)

Whole-body distribution of FCH shows no particular differences compared to the distribution of 11C-choline.[35] Physiologic increased tracer uptake accumulation is present in different tissues for all radiolabeled choline PET tracers—mainly in the liver, spleen, pancreas, and other exocrine organs (**Fig. 2**). Wyss and colleagues[36] reported that FCH uptake can be seen in inflammatory soft tissues in an animal model. This inflammation may be the cause of bilateral mild FCH uptake that is sometimes seen in inguinal lymph nodes.[35] Degenerative bone lesions usually do not show abnormal FCH uptake; however, it is noted that nonspecific inflammatory changes may cause mildly increased FCH uptake in intervertebral joints.[37] Recent fractures also show positive FCH uptake (**Fig. 3**).[37]

Some studies have suggested that the accuracy of FCH is comparable to that of 11C-choline;[38,39] however, to the authors' knowledge, to date, no comparative data are available.

The major advantage of 18F-choline versus 11C-choline radiotracer is the longer half-life of FCH, which provides the distribution of this tracer to PET institutions without an on-site cyclotron. Furthermore, the longer half-life of FCH allows performing delayed images, which may improve the specificity of PET studies.[40–42] 11C-choline, however, has low renal excretion, which in turn increases the accuracy of PET imaging in the evaluation of the pelvis. On the other hand, 18F-choline radiotracers show significant urinary excretion. It has been suggested that early urinary appearance of 18F-choline compounds is caused by incomplete tubular reabsorption of intact tracer or by enhanced excretion of oxidized metabolites.[26]

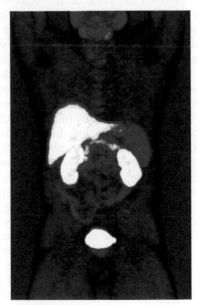

Fig. 2. 18F-choline distribution: increased tracer uptake in the liver, spleen, pancreas, and salivary glands; mild diffuse uptake in gastrointestinal tract.

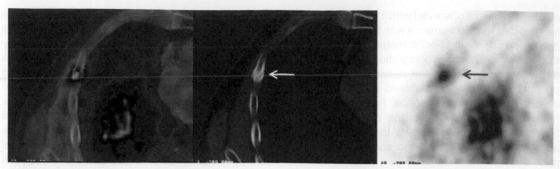

Fig. 3. Rib fracture with positive 18F-choline uptake seen in PET study (*red arrow*) correlated with morphologic change on CT (*white arrow*).

STAGING
Primary Tumor

The ability of noninvasive diagnostic imaging modalities to delineate prostate cancer tissue from normal prostate, benign prostate hyperplasia (BPH), and focal chronic prostatitis is of great concern. 11C-choline was first introduced by Hara and coworkers[30,43–45] for the imaging of different malignancies, particularly brain and prostate cancers. Sutinen and colleagues[46] evaluated the association between the uptake of 11C-choline and the histologic grade of malignancy, Gleason score, volume of the prostate, and prostate-specific antigen (PSA). They could not demonstrate any association between prostate cancer aggressiveness (as depicted by the differentiation grade or Gleason score) and uptake of 11C-choline. There was also no association between serum PSA value or the volume of the prostate and the uptake of 11C-choline. Moreover, the difference between the standardized uptake value (SUV) of prostate cancer and BPH was not significant in that study.

In a recent study, however, Reske and colleagues[47] showed a clear differentiation between prostate cancer and benign processes (BPH or chronic prostatitis) by means of SUV using 11C-choline PET-CT imaging. In that study, the maximum SUV correlated significantly with T stage but not with PSA or Gleason score.

In another study, the in vivo uptake of 11C-choline with PET was correlated with cell proliferation in human prostate cancer.[48] No significant correlation between SUV of choline and Ki-67 expression (as a marker of proliferation) or tumor grade was found. Recently, Giovacchini and colleagues[49] reported that 11C-choline is not suitable for the initial diagnosis and local staging of prostate cancer but it could be used to monitor the response to antiandrogen therapy, although this has been disputed by other reports.[50,51]

Recent successful labeling of choline compounds with 18F introduced FECH and FCH as two 18F-choline tracers that are currently used in PET imaging.[25,26,28,29] Some studies reported that the differentiation of BPH from cancerous prostate lesions is also not possible with FCH PET-CT.[35,52] In a recent study by the authors' group[52] of a relatively large population of intermediate- and high-risk prostate cancer patients, however, good agreement (81%) was found between regions with maximum FCH uptake on PET and sextants with maximum tumoral involvement in the histopathologic examinations, which can be helpful in guiding biopsy (**Fig. 4**).

Kwee and colleagues[53] evaluated the suitability of delayed or dual-phase FCH PET for localizing malignancy in the prostate gland. They found that malignant areas in prostate consistently demonstrate stable or increasing FCH uptake, whereas most areas containing benign tissues showed decreasing uptake. They concluded that delayed or dual-phase imaging after injection of FCH may improve the performance of FCH PET for localizing malignant areas of the prostate. This pattern, however, was not seen in recent studies performed by the authors' group[52] or by Cimitan and colleagues.[41]

Lymph Node Metastases (N Stage)

Lymph node metastases are detected in about 25% of prostate cancer patients depending on the tumor stage and grade.[54,55] The presence of lymph node metastases is correlated with progressive disease and subsequently decreases the 5-year disease-free survival rate from 85% in nonmetastatic patients to approximately 50% for pN1 disease.[54] Therefore, accurate identification of tumor infiltration in regional lymph nodes is of key importance for implications on treatment strategy during the operation and on the initiation of adjuvant therapy regimens.[56] Pelvic lymphadenectomy is still the gold standard for lymph node

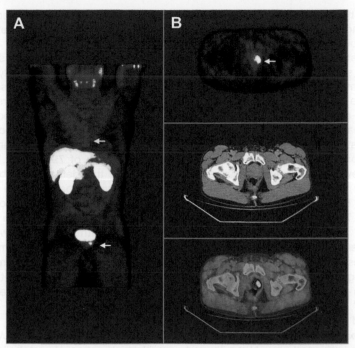

Fig. 4. 18F-choline PET-CT in preoperative evaluation of an intermediate-risk prostate cancer patient. (*A*) Maximum-intensity processing (MIP) image: focal tracer uptake in the left part of prostate (*white arrow*). Inflammatory soft tissue uptake seen in esophagus (*yellow arrow*), suggestive of esophagitis. (*B*) Transaxial images: focal increased tracer 18F-choline uptake in the left mid part of prostate (*white arrow*) consistent with prostate cancer.

staging in prostate cancer; however, this invasive procedure has its own limitations and is associated with morbidity.[57–59] Since nodal involvement is not always correlated with enlargement, conventional imaging modalities such as CT and MR imaging have limited sensitivity in determining malignant lymph nodes in prostate cancer.[60–62]

De Jong and colleagues[63] showed promising results with 11C-choline PET in the preoperative lymph node staging of 67 newly diagnosed prostate cancer patients, with a sensitivity of 80% in patient-based analysis. It should be noted, however, that a mean PSA level of 123 ng/mL may induce a referral bias in that study. In a recent publication, Hacker and colleagues[9] reported a lower sensitivity of FCH PET-CT (10%) when comparing sentinel node dissection (80%) in 20 patients who had intermediate- and high-risk of extraglandular disease and concluded that FCH PET-CT is not useful for detection of occult lymph node metastases. It is important to mention that the mean diameter of metastatic lymph nodes in that study was 3.8 mm, which is less than spatial resolution of the PET scanner (ie, ~4.8 mm). Moreover, a large FCH-positive (ie, 25-mm diameter) malignant pelvic lymph node was a false negative on sentinel lymph dissection.

Schiavina and colleagues[13] recently evaluated the accuracy of 11C-choline PET-CT for preoperative lymph node staging in 57 intermediate- and high-risk prostate cancer patients and compared it with two currently used nomograms. They showed that 11C-choline PET-CT performed better than clinical nomograms for the detection of lymph node metastases, with equal sensitivity (60%) and better specificity.

In a recent study from the authors' group, FCH PET-CT showed an overall sensitivity of 45%, specificity of 96%, positive predictive value (PPV) of 82%, and negative predictive value (NPV) of 83% for the detection of lymph node metastases.[52] Nevertheless, in lymph nodes larger than 5 mm, the sensitivity, specificity, PPV, and NPV were 66%, 96%, 82%, and 92%, respectively. As expected, FCH PET-CT showed limited value in the detection of micro and lymph node metastases smaller than 5 mm. The failure to detect the small metastases in the lymph nodes could be due to the limited resolution of the current generations of PET scanners, which is about 4.8 mm.

Bone Metastases (M Stage)

Although prostate cancer is one of the few cancers that grows so slowly that it may never be life threatening, it can show an aggressive pattern and may spread, causing the death of patients mainly due to metastatic bone disease. Therefore, early diagnosis of metastatic bone involvement is of key importance for selecting appropriate therapy, to assess the patient's prognosis, and to evaluate the efficacy of bone-specific treatments that may reduce future bone-associated morbidity.

Cimitan and colleagues[41] examined the value of FCH PET-CT in postoperative assessment of 100 prostate cancer patients who had persistent raised serum PSA levels, suggestive of local recurrences or distant metastases. FCH PET-CT correctly detected bone metastases in 21% of patients; however, 76% of them were receiving hormone therapy. They concluded that FCH uptake in bone seems to be highly predictive of skeletal metastases; however, in the authors' opinion, this finding should be interpreted with caution in patients who are being treated with hormone therapy.[64]

The evaluation of 111 patients (43 patients for staging and 68 patients for restaging) using FCH PET-CT was reported by Husarik and colleagues.[42] Pathologic FCH accumulation in osseous structures was seen in about 15% of patients and was subsequently confirmed by bone scan, MR imaging, and CT morphology.

These investigators concluded that FCH PET-CT is well able to depict bone metastases in prostate cancer patients.

In a recent prospective study, the authors' group examined the capability of FCH PET-CT to detect metastatic bone disease in prostate cancer in 70 patients and, for the first time, used CT to assess the pattern of metabolic uptake by FCH in relation to morphologic changes in bone.[37] FCH PET-CT showed a sensitivity, specificity, and accuracy of 79%, 97%, and 84%, respectively, for the detection of bone metastases in prostate cancer patients. The authors' group also observed a dynamic and progressive pattern of abnormality associated with bone metastases: beginning with bone marrow involvement, then generally osteoblastic but sometimes osteoclastic changes, and finally progressing to densely sclerotic lesions without metabolic activity.[65] In addition, FCH PET-CT showed promising results for the early detection of bone metastases. Furthermore, the authors' group found that a Hounsfield units level of above 825 is associated with an absence of metabolic activity with FCH. Almost all of the FCH-negative sclerotic lesions were detected in patients who were undergoing hormone therapy, which raises the possibility that these lesions may no longer be viable. This

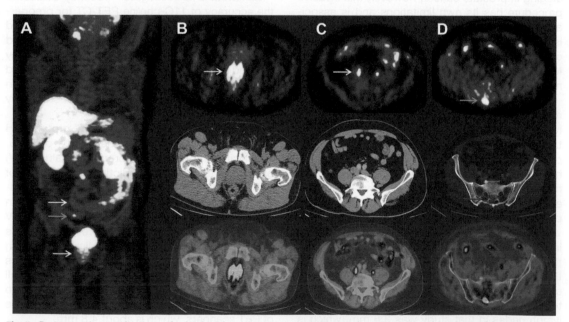

Fig. 5. Preoperative evaluation of a high-risk prostate cancer patient who was primarily upstaged by 18F-choline PET-CT. (*A*) MIP image (for explanation of arrows, see Fig. 5B–D). (*B*) Transaxial PET-CT images with intensive tracer uptake in the prostate (*yellow arrow*). (*C*) Transaxial PET-CT images with abnormal increased tracer uptake in a malignant pelvic lymph node (*white arrow*). (*D*) Transaxial PET-CT images with focal abnormal tracer uptake in sacrum (*blue arrow*) without significant morphologic change on CT (*red arrow*) due to bone marrow metastasis.

pattern, however, should be further clarified in future studies. Finally, in metastatic bone lesions, a significant increase of FCH uptake was seen in the late images (ie, about 110 minutes post injection). This finding confirmed the previous data reported by the authors' group[10,40,64,66] and in other similar studies.[41,42]

Therapeutic Management

Different treatment options, consisting of watchful waiting, radical prostatectomy, radiotherapy, antiandrogen therapy, or a combination of these, may be considered depending on the clinical stage of the prostate cancer patient. Thus, accurate staging of the disease has an important role in the determination of subsequent therapeutic approaches. Bone scintigraphy and CT are routinely used for preoperative staging of bone and lymph node status in high-risk prostate cancer patients. CT, however, has low accuracy in the detection of lymph node metastases, and bone scanning suffers from low specificity and has limited value in the detection of early marrow-based disease.[67]

In a recent study by the authors' group, FCH PET-CT led to a change in the therapeutic management of 15% of the patient population due to the detection of lymph node metastases, bone metastases, or both.[52] All but two patients belonged to the high-risk group. In this high-risk group, 20% of patients were upstaged by FCH PET-CT, thus changing the therapy consequence from operative to nonoperative management (**Fig. 5**).

RESTAGING

Prostate cancer disease is generally monitored by PSA after initial therapy. Persistent increase in PSA level after treatment suggests biochemical recurrence of disease. About 27% to 53% of prostate cancer patients develop biochemical recurrence up to 10 years after radical prostatectomy, and 16% to 35% of patients receive second-line therapy within 5 years after initial treatment.[68] An increase in PSA level to more than 0.2 ng/mL after surgery can be used as a practical cutoff value for diagnosis of local

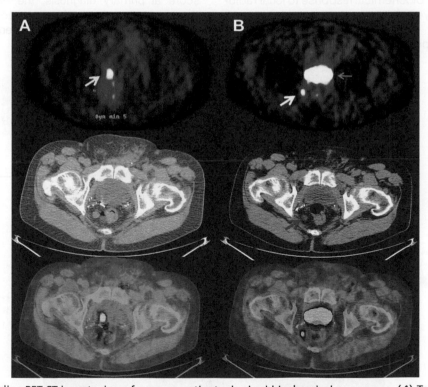

Fig. 6. 18F-choline PET-CT in restaging of a cancer patient who had biochemical recurrence. (*A*) Tansaxial PET-CT dynamic pelvic images (5 minutes post injection): intensive focal 18F-choline uptake in the right prostate bed (*yellow arrow*) suggestive of local recurrence. (*B*) Tansaxial PET-CT pelvic images (15 minutes post injection): focal abnormal tracer uptake in right perirectal region (*white arrow*) with morphologic correlation on CT (*red arrow*). Rapid urinary excretion of 18F-choline is also noted about 15 minutes after tracer administration with tracer accumulation in the bladder (*blue arrow*).

recurrence of prostate cancer.[69–72] Of the patients who develop biochemical relapse, 50% show only isolated local recurrence and the other 50% show distant metastases with or without local recurrence.[70,71,73] Therefore, accurate diagnosis of local recurrence is highly desirable because treatment approaches and outcome of local or disseminated disease are basically different. Conventional imaging modalities such as transrectal ultrasonography, MR imaging, CT, bone scan, and immunoscintigraphy with 111In-capromab pendetide are not sensitive enough to detect metastatic or recurrent prostate cancer.[74–80]

In some recent studies, the value of PET-CT imaging using 11C-choline[51,72] and FCH[42] in the detection of recurrent prostate cancer was evaluated.

Reske and colleagues[72] studied 49 patients who had prostate adenocarcinoma after radical prostatectomy with occult relapse. 11C-choline PET-CT showed a sensitivity and specificity of 73% and 88%, respectively, in the detection of local recurrence in prostate cancer. In addition, 11C-choline PET-CT was able to identify 71% of patients who had favorable biochemical response to local radiotherapy at 2-year follow-up.

In another study, Krause and colleagues[51] showed a positive relationship between the detection rate of 11C-choline PET-CT and serum PSA levels in patients who had biochemical recurrence of prostate cancer after initial treatment. The detection rate of 11C-choline ranged from 36% for a PSA level below 1 ng/mL to 73% for a PSA value 3 ng/mL or higher, which allows not only to diagnose but also to localize recurrent disease, with implications on therapeutic management (localized versus systemic therapy). Husarik and colleagues[42] examined the value of FCH PET-CT in the detection of recurrent prostate cancer diseases and showed similar results, with sensitivities of 71% at PSA levels lower than 2 ng/mL and 86% at any PSA level (Fig. 6). Data from Cimitan and colleagues'[41] study of a large sample of postoperative prostate cancer patients, however, suggested that FCH PET-CT has no significant impact in therapeutic care of prostate cancer patients who have biochemical recurrence until the PSA level increases above 4 ng/mL. In the authors' opinion, the PSA level is not the only parameter that defines the presence or absence of FCH uptake. Other factors, such as the initial grade of disease, the PSA level and the Gleason score at primary diagnosis, the PSA doubling time, and the time to recurrence after initial therapy, may also have an influence on FCH uptake.

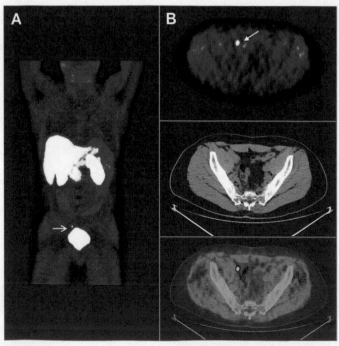

Fig. 7. 18F-choline PET-CT in postoperative evaluation of a prostate cancer patient under antiandrogen treatment. (A) MIP image: focal abnormal tracer uptake in right pelvis (*yellow arrow*). (B) Transaxial PET-CT images from pelvis with intensive focal 18F-choline in the right external iliac region suggestive of malignant lymph node (*white arrow*).

INFLUENCE OF HORMONE THERAPY

Similar to FDG,[10] it may be assumed that choline uptake under hormone therapy or chemotherapy will be reduced. In patients who have already received hormone therapy, the magnitude of the PSA level is likely to be suppressed and may not correlate well with tumor size or metabolism. Krause and colleagues[51] evaluated 63 prostate cancer patients who had biochemical recurrence after initial treatment by 11C-choline PET-CT, of whom 17 patients were receiving hormone therapy. They found that antiandrogen therapy had no significant effect on the detection rate of 11C-choline PET-CT. Nevertheless, there are reports of choline uptake decreasing after initiating hormone therapy;[81] the authors do not know, however, whether the influence on choline metabolism and on PSA level occurs in parallel. It cannot be ruled out that the FCH PET signal is influenced less strongly than the PSA level.

Although De Jong and colleagues[63] raised the question of whether the use of FCH PET after initial therapy should be restricted to patients who have a PSA level higher than 5 ng/mL, the authors were able to show in a former study by their group that FCH PET-CT should not be limited to PSA values below 5.0 ng/mL.[82] Moreover, the authors believe that in patients undergoing hormone therapy (and who have PSA levels < 5.0 ng/mL), FCH PET-CT can also provide additional information concerning pathologic lesions (**Fig. 7**).

SUMMARY

The accuracy and biodistribution of 18F-choline seems to be comparable to that of 11C-choline used in PET imaging for the assessment of prostate cancer.

Radiolabeled-choline PET can be useful in guiding biopsy for the assessment of primary prostate cancer; however, it cannot accurately differentiate BPH or chronic prostatitis from cancerous prostate lesions by means of SUV.

In the detection of micro and lymph node metastases smaller than 5 mm, radiolabeled-choline PET-CT seems to have limited value. The failure to detect the small metastases in the lymph nodes could be due to the limited resolution of the current generations of PET scanners; however, it should be mentioned that all other current radiologic modalities and clinical staging nomograms also have limited diagnostic performance for N staging.

PET imaging using radiolabeled choline showed promising results in the detection of bone metastases, especially early marrow-based disease in prostate cancer patients.

Radiolabeled choline seems to have the potential in primary staging of high-risk prostate cancer patients to exclude distant metastases when surgical treatment is planned. PET-CT imaging using radiolabeled choline has proved to play a significant diagnostic role in the assessment of recurrent disease after initial treatment.

Finally, on the basis of current data, the authors believe that proper clinical indication is of key importance for referring prostate cancer patients to metabolic PET imaging using radiolabeled choline.

REFERENCES

1. Effert PJ, Bares R, Handt S, et al. Metabolic imaging of untreated prostate cancer by positron emission tomography with 18fluorine-labeled deoxyglucose. J Urol 1996;155(3):994–8.
2. Heicappell R, Muller-Mattheis V, Reinhardt M, et al. Staging of pelvic lymph nodes in neoplasms of the bladder and prostate by positron emission tomography with 2-[(18)F]-2-deoxy-D-glucose. Eur Urol 1999;36(6):582–7.
3. Hofer C, Laubenbacher C, Block T, et al. Fluorine-18-fluorodeoxyglucose positron emission tomography is useless for the detection of local recurrence after radical prostatectomy. Eur Urol 1999;36(1):31–5.
4. Liu IJ, Zafar MB, Lai YH, et al. Fluorodeoxyglucose positron emission tomography studies in diagnosis and staging of clinically organ-confined prostate cancer. Urology 2001;57(1):108–11.
5. Morris MJ, Akhurst T, Osman I, et al. Fluorinated deoxyglucose positron emission tomography imaging in progressive metastatic prostate cancer. Urology 2002;59(6):913–8.
6. Shreve PD, Grossman HB, Gross MD, et al. Metastatic prostate cancer: initial findings of PET with 2-deoxy-2-[F-18]fluoro-D-glucose. Radiology 1996;199(3):751–6.
7. Kumar R, Zhuang H, Alavi A. PET in the management of urologic malignancies. Radiol Clin North Am 2004;42(6):1141–53, ix.
8. Testa C, Schiavina R, Lodi R, et al. Prostate cancer: sextant localization with MR imaging, MR spectroscopy, and 11C-choline PET/CT. Radiology 2007;244(3):797–806.
9. Hacker A, Jeschke S, Leeb K, et al. Detection of pelvic lymph node metastases in patients with clinically localized prostate cancer: comparison of [18F]fluorocholine positron emission tomography-computerized tomography and laparoscopic radio-isotope guided sentinel lymph node dissection. J Urol 2006;176(5):2014–8 [discussion: 2018–9].
10. Langsteger W, Heinisch M, Fogelman I. The role of fluorodeoxyglucose, 18F-dihydroxyphenylalanine,

18F-choline, and 18F-fluoride in bone imaging with emphasis on prostate and breast. Semin Nucl Med 2006;36(1):73–92.

11. Scher B, Seitz M, Albinger W, et al. Value of 11C-choline PET and PET/CT in patients with suspected prostate cancer. Eur J Nucl Med Mol Imaging 2007;34(1):45–53.

12. Hricak H, Choyke PL, Eberhardt SC, et al. Imaging prostate cancer: a multidisciplinary perspective. Radiology 2007;243(1):28–53.

13. Schiavina R, Scattoni V, Castellucci P, et al. 11C-choline positron emission tomography/computerized tomography for preoperative lymph-node staging in intermediate-risk and high-risk prostate cancer: comparison with clinical staging nomograms. Eur Urol 2008;54(2):392–401.

14. Zeisel SH. Dietary choline: biochemistry, physiology, and pharmacology. Annu Rev Nutr 1981;1: 95–121.

15. Roivainen A, Forsback S, Gronroos T, et al. Blood metabolism of [methyl-11C]choline; implications for in vivo imaging with positron emission tomography. Eur J Nucl Med 2000;27(1):25–32.

16. Ishidate K. Choline/ethanolamine kinase from mammalian tissues. Biochim Biophys Acta 1997; 1348(1–2):70–8.

17. Wright PS, Morand JN, Kent C. Regulation of phosphatidylcholine biosynthesis in Chinese hamster ovary cells by reversible membrane association of CTP: phosphocholine cytidylyltransferase. J Biol Chem 1985;260(13):7919–26.

18. Wettstein M, Weik C, Holneicher C, et al. Betaine as an osmolyte in rat liver: metabolism and cell-to-cell interactions. Hepatology 1998;27(3):787–93.

19. Wajda IJ, Manigault I, Hudick JP, et al. Regional and subcellular distribution of choline acetyltransferase in the brain of rats. J Neurochem 1973;21(6): 1385–401.

20. Katz-Brull R, Degani H. Kinetics of choline transport and phosphorylation in human breast cancer cells; NMR application of the zero trans method. Anticancer Res 1996;16(3B):1375–80.

21. Zeisel SH. Choline phospholipids: signal transduction and carcinogenesis. FASEB J 1993;7(6): 551–7.

22. Wald LL, Nelson SJ, Day MR, et al. Serial proton magnetic resonance spectroscopy imaging of glioblastoma multiforme after brachytherapy. J Neurosurg 1997;87(4):525–34.

23. Tedeschi G, Lundbom N, Raman R, et al. Increased choline signal coinciding with malignant degeneration of cerebral gliomas: a serial proton magnetic resonance spectroscopy imaging study. J Neurosurg 1997;87(4):516–24.

24. Miller BL, Chang L, Booth R, et al. In vivo 1H MRS choline. Correlation with in vitro chemistry/histology. Life Sci 1996;58(22):1929–35.

25. Hara T, Kosaka N, Kishi H. Development of (18)F-fluoroethylcholine for cancer imaging with PET: synthesis, biochemistry, and prostate cancer imaging. J Nucl Med 2002;43(2):187–99.

26. DeGrado TR, Coleman RE, Wang S, et al. Synthesis and evaluation of 18F-labeled choline as an oncologic tracer for positron emission tomography: initial findings in prostate cancer. Cancer Res 2001;61(1): 110–7.

27. Bender H, Wiludda V, Matthies A, et al. Use of 18F-fluoro-ethyl- and methyl-choline PET in prostate cancer: a comparative and feasibility study. Presented at the 44th meeting of the German Society of Nuclear Medicine 2006.

28. DeGrado TR, Reiman RE, Price DT, et al. Pharmacokinetics and radiation dosimetry of 18F-fluorocholine. J Nucl Med 2002;43(1):92–6.

29. DeGrado TR, Baldwin SW, Wang S, et al. Synthesis and evaluation of (18)F-labeled choline analogs as oncologic PET tracers. J Nucl Med 2001;42(12): 1805–14.

30. Hara T, Kosaka N, Kishi H. PET imaging of prostate cancer using carbon-11-choline. J Nucl Med 1998; 39(6):990–5.

31. Pascali C, Bogni A, Iwata R, et al. [11C]Methylation on a Sep-Pak cartridge: a convenient way to produce [N-methyl-11C]choline. J Labelled Comp Radiopharm 2000;43:195–203.

32. Langsteger W, Beheshti M, Vali R, et al. Prostate cancer. In: Bombardieri E, Buscombe J, Lucignani G, editors. Advances in nuclear oncology. 1st edition. London: Informa healthcare; 2007. p. 109–31.

33. Iwata R, Pascali C, Bogni A, et al. [18F]fluoromethyl triflate, a novel and reactive [18F]fluoromethylating agent: preparation and application to the on-column preparation of [18F]fluorocholine. Appl Radiat Isot 2002;57(3):347–52.

34. Nader M, Hoepping A. Metamorphosis of a dedicated FDG disposable kit module to a multipurpose synthesizer [abstract]. Nuklearmedizin 2005;44: A192, 197.

35. Schmid DT, John H, Zweifel R, et al. Fluorocholine PET/CT in patients with prostate cancer: initial experience. Radiology 2005;235(2):623–8.

36. Wyss MT, Weber B, Honer M, et al. 18F-choline in experimental soft tissue infection assessed with autoradiography and high-resolution PET. Eur J Nucl Med Mol Imaging 2004;31(3):312–6.

37. Beheshti M, Vali R, Waldenberger P, et al. The use of F-18 choline PET in the assessment of bone metastases in prostate cancer: correlation with morphological changes on CT. Mol Imaging Biol Mar 27 2009 [epub ahead of print].

38. Hara T, Kondo T, Kosaka N. Use of 18F-choline and 11C-choline as contrast agents in positron emission tomography imaging-guided stereotactic biopsy sampling of gliomas. J Neurosurg 2003;99(3):474–9.

39. Nanni C, Castellucci P, Farsad M, et al. 11C/18F-choline PET or 11C/18F-acetate PET in prostate cancer: may a choice be recommended? Eur J Nucl Med Mol Imaging 2007;34(10):1704–5.

40. Beheshti M, Haim S, Nader M, et al. Assessment of bone metastases in patients with prostate cancer by dual-phase F-18 fluor choline PET/CT. Eur J Nucl Med Mol Imaging 2006;33(Suppl 2):208.

41. Cimitan M, Bortolus R, Morassut S, et al. [18F]fluorocholine PET/CT imaging for the detection of recurrent prostate cancer at PSA relapse: experience in 100 consecutive patients. Eur J Nucl Med Mol Imaging 2006;33(12):1387–98.

42. Husarik DB, Miralbell R, Dubs M, et al. Evaluation of [(18)F]-choline PET/CT for staging and restaging of prostate cancer. Eur J Nucl Med Mol Imaging 2008;35(2):253–63.

43. Hara T, Kosaka N, Shinoura N, et al. PET imaging of brain tumor with [methyl-11C]choline. J Nucl Med 1997;38(6):842–7.

44. Hara T, Inagaki K, Kosaka N, et al. Sensitive detection of mediastinal lymph node metastasis of lung cancer with 11C-choline PET. J Nucl Med 2000; 41(9):1507–13.

45. Kobori O, Kirihara Y, Kosaka N, et al. Positron emission tomography of esophageal carcinoma using (11)C-choline and (18)F-fluorodeoxyglucose: a novel method of preoperative lymph node staging. Cancer 1999;86(9):1638–48.

46. Sutinen E, Nurmi M, Roivainen A, et al. Kinetics of [(11)C]choline uptake in prostate cancer: a PET study. Eur J Nucl Med Mol Imaging 2004;31(3):317–24.

47. Reske SN, Blumstein NM, Neumaier B, et al. Imaging prostate cancer with 11C-choline PET/CT. J Nucl Med 2006;47(8):1249–54.

48. Breeuwsma AJ, Pruim J, Jongen MM, et al. In vivo uptake of [11C]choline does not correlate with cell proliferation in human prostate cancer. Eur J Nucl Med Mol Imaging 2005;32(6):668–73.

49. Giovacchini G, Picchio M, Coradeschi E, et al. [(11)C]choline uptake with PET/CT for the initial diagnosis of prostate cancer: relation to PSA levels, tumour stage and anti-androgenic therapy. Eur J Nucl Med Mol Imaging 2008;35(6):1065–73.

50. Jadvar H, Gurbuz A, Li X, et al. Choline autoradiography of human prostate cancer xenograft: effect of castration. Mol Imaging 2008;7(3):147–52.

51. Krause BJ, Souvatzoglou M, Tuncel M, et al. The detection rate of [11C]choline-PET/CT depends on the serum PSA-value in patients with biochemical recurrence of prostate cancer. Eur J Nucl Med Mol Imaging 2008;35(1):18–23.

52. Beheshti M, Imamovic L, Broinger G, et al. F-18 Choline PET-CT in the preoperative staging of prostate cancer patients with intermediate and high risk of extra-capsular disease: a prospective study in 130 patients. J Nucl Med 2009;50(Suppl 1).

53. Kwee SA, Wei H, Sesterhenn I, et al. Localization of primary prostate cancer with dual-phase 18F-fluorocholine PET. J Nucl Med 2006;47(2):262–9.

54. Danella JF, deKernion JB, Smith RB, et al. The contemporary incidence of lymph node metastases in prostate cancer: implications for laparoscopic lymph node dissection. J Urol 1993; 149(6):1488–91.

55. Partin AW, Mangold LA, Lamm DM, et al. Contemporary update of prostate cancer staging nomograms (Partin tables) for the new millennium. Urology 2001;58(6):843–8.

56. Messing EM, Manola J, Sarosdy M, et al. Immediate hormonal therapy compared with observation after radical prostatectomy and pelvic lymphadenectomy in men with node-positive prostate cancer. N Engl J Med 1999;341(24):1781–8.

57. Bratt O, Elfving P, Flodgren P, et al. Morbidity of pelvic lymphadenectomy, radical retropubic prostatectomy and external radiotherapy in patients with localised prostatic cancer. Scand J Urol Nephrol 1994;28(3):265–71.

58. Paul DB, Loening SA, Narayana AS, et al. Morbidity from pelvic lymphadenectomy in staging carcinoma of the prostate. J Urol 1983;129(6):1141–4.

59. Briganti A, Chun FK, Salonia A, et al. Complications and other surgical outcomes associated with extended pelvic lymphadenectomy in men with localized prostate cancer. Eur Urol 2006;50(5): 1006–13.

60. Hricak H, Dooms GC, Jeffrey RB, et al. Prostatic carcinoma: staging by clinical assessment, CT, and MR imaging. Radiology 1987;162(2):331–6.

61. Platt JF, Bree RL, Schwab RE. The accuracy of CT in the staging of carcinoma of the prostate. AJR Am J Roentgenol 1987;149(2):315–8.

62. Jager GJ, Barentsz JO, Oosterhof GO, et al. Pelvic adenopathy in prostatic and urinary bladder carcinoma: MR imaging with a three-dimensional TI-weighted magnetization-prepared rapid gradient-echo sequence. AJR Am J Roentgenol 1996;167(6):1503–7.

63. De Jong IJ, Pruim J, Elsinga PH, et al. Preoperative staging of pelvic lymph nodes in prostate cancer by 11C-choline PET. J Nucl Med 2003; 44(3):331–5.

64. Beheshti M, Vali R, Langsteger W. [18F]fluorocholine PET/CT in the assessment of bone metastases in prostate cancer. Eur J Nucl Med Mol Imaging 2007;34(8):1316–7 [author reply 1318–9].

65. Beheshti M, Langsteger W, Fogelman I. Prostate cancer: role of SPECT and PET in imaging bone metastases. Semin Nucl Med 2009, in press.

66. Langsteger W, Beheshti M, Pöcher S, et al. Fluor Choline (FCH) PET-CT in preoperative staging and follow up of prostate cancer. Mol Imaging Biol 2006;8:69.

67. Purohit RS, Shinohara K, Meng MV, et al. Imaging clinically localized prostate cancer. Urol Clin North Am 2003;30(2):279–93.
68. Bott SR. Management of recurrent disease after radical prostatectomy. Prostate Cancer Prostatic Dis 2004;7(3):211–6.
69. Boccon-Gibod L, Djavan WB, Hammerer P, et al. Management of prostate-specific antigen relapse in prostate cancer: a European Consensus. Int J Clin Pract 2004;58(4):382–90.
70. Pound CR, Partin AW, Epstein JI, et al. Prostate-specific antigen after anatomic radical retropubic prostatectomy. Patterns of recurrence and cancer control. Urol Clin North Am 1997;24(2):395–406.
71. Cox JD, Gallagher MJ, Hammond EH, et al. Consensus statements on radiation therapy of prostate cancer: guidelines for prostate re-biopsy after radiation and for radiation therapy with rising prostate-specific antigen levels after radical prostatectomy. American Society for Therapeutic Radiology and Oncology Consensus Panel. J Clin Oncol 1999;17(4):1155.
72. Reske SN, Blumstein NM, Glatting G. [11C]choline PET/CT imaging in occult local relapse of prostate cancer after radical prostatectomy. Eur J Nucl Med Mol Imaging 2008;35(1):9–17.
73. Pound CR, Partin AW, Eisenberger MA, et al. Natural history of progression after PSA elevation following radical prostatectomy. JAMA 1999;281(17):1591–7.
74. Hricak H, Schoder H, Pucar D, et al. Advances in imaging in the postoperative patient with a rising prostate-specific antigen level. Semin Oncol 2003; 30(5):616–34.

75. Kurhanewicz J, Vigneron DB, Males RG, et al. The prostate: MR imaging and spectroscopy. Present and future. Radiol Clin North Am 2000;38(1): 115–38, viii–ix.
76. May F, Treumann T, Dettmar P, et al. Limited value of endorectal magnetic resonance imaging and transrectal ultrasonography in the staging of clinically localized prostate cancer. BJU Int 2001;87(1):66–9.
77. Nudell DM, Wefer AE, Hricak H, et al. Imaging for recurrent prostate cancer. Radiol Clin North Am 2000;38(1):213–29.
78. Parivar F, Hricak H, Shinohara K, et al. Detection of locally recurrent prostate cancer after cryosurgery: evaluation by transrectal ultrasound, magnetic resonance imaging, and three-dimensional proton magnetic resonance spectroscopy. Urology 1996; 48(4):594–9.
79. Smith PH, Bono A, Calais da Silva F, et al. Some limitations of the radioisotope bone scan in patients with metastatic prostatic cancer. A subanalysis of EORTC trial 30853. The EORTC Urological Group. Cancer 1990;66(5 Suppl):1009–16.
80. Yu KK, Hricak H. Imaging prostate cancer. Radiol Clin North Am 2000;38(1):59–85, viii.
81. Coleman R, DeGrado T, Wang S, et al. 9:30–9:45. Preliminary evaluation of F-18 fluorocholine (FCH) as a PET tumor imaging agent. Clin Positron Imaging 2000;3(4):147.
82. Heinisch M, Dirisamer A, Loidl W, et al. Positron emission tomography/computed tomography with F-18-fluorocholine for restaging of prostate cancer patients: meaningful at PSA< 5ng/ml? Mol Imaging Biol 2006;8(1):43–8.

PET Imaging of Prostate Cancer: Other Tracers

Eric M. Rohren, MD, PhD*, Homer A. Macapinlac, MD

KEYWORDS

- Prostate cancer • PET/CT • Methionine
- Testosterone derivatives • Androgen receptors • Hypoxia

There are significant limitations in the current options for imaging of patients with prostate carcinoma.[1–10] It is recognized that there is a need for development of new imaging modalities and tracers for detection, characterization, staging, and re-staging of prostate cancer. Although fluorodeoxyglucose (FDG) is the mainstay of clinical imaging, many other isotope and tracer combinations can be imaged with PET. Several of these non-FDG tracers hold promise for evaluation of prostatic malignancies and other genitourinary tumors. The most often studied non-FDG compounds in prostate cancer are choline tracers (C-11 choline and F-18 fluorocholine) and acetate tracers (C-11 acetate and F-18 fluoroacetate). As discussed in other articles within this issue, these agents overcome some of the limitations of FDG in the imaging of prostate tumors.

One of the strengths of nuclear imaging lies in the variety of radiotracers capable of being imaged. In the last 15 years, various compounds other than FDG, choline, and acetate have been studied in the hope of identifying the ideal imaging agent for prostate cancer. Although none has entered clinical practice, important lessons have been learned in the process, and the understanding of the biology and natural history of prostate malignancy has been expanded. In this article, the use of imaging agents other than FDG, choline, and acetate is discussed.

PET IMAGING USING AMINO ACID DERIVATIVES

Localization and uptake of radiolabeled amino acid derivatives have been used as means to image many tumor types. The specific localization of amino acid radiotracers occurs primarily via intracellular localization through receptor-mediated uptake. Once inside the cell, some of these agents proceed through protein catabolism, but this is thought to be a minor contributor in terms of imaging. Numerous studies have been performed using amino acid tracers in the evaluation of brain tumors, and a significant number of research articles have examined the role of these tracers in patients with sarcoma. The extent of literature in prostate cancer is smaller, but amino acid tracers have shown some promise.

The most studied amino acid tracer in prostate carcinoma is L-[1-^{11}C]-methionine. Uptake and accumulation of this tracer in tumor cells indirectly reflects amino acid metabolism and transport.[11,12] The agent is actively transported into the cytosol from plasma by an Na+ dependent membrane transporter system. There are several potential advantages to using ^{11}C-methionine as a PET imaging tracer for evaluation of the prostate gland and pelvis (**Fig. 1**). The first advantage is that there is rapid serum clearance of radiotracer followed by relatively steady state of plasma activity. Methionine is metabolized in the liver and pancreas with little to no renal excretion, which makes evaluation of the prostate gland and other pelvic structures easier than with tracers that have a high degree of urinary excretion, such as FDG. Finally, with specific regards to the prostate gland, the elevated expression of cell surface transporters in malignancies of the prostate gland results in uptake and high intracellular concentration of methionine. The expression of these transporters is lower in normal prostate tissue and in regions of benign prostatic hypertrophy and prostatitis.

In an early study of 12 patients with androgen-independent prostate cancer,[13] all sites of known osseous and extraosseous tumor that were visualized by bone scintigraphy and standard

U.T. M. D. Anderson Cancer Center, 1515 Holcombe Boulevard, Unit 1264, Houston, TX 77030, USA
* Corresponding author.
E-mail address: eric.rohren@mdanderson.org (E.M. Rohren).

PET Clin 4 (2009) 185–192
doi:10.1016/j.cpet.2009.05.004

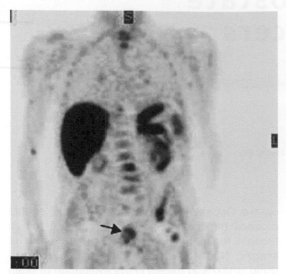

Fig. 1. Coronal view of an ^{11}C-methionine PET scan in a patient with metastatic prostate cancer shows recurrent disease in the pelvis (*arrow*) and multiple sites of osseous metastatic disease.

cross-sectional imaging were identified on ^{11}C-methionine PET scanning. A subsequent study[14] examined 10 patients with histologically confirmed prostate adenocarcinoma and documented disease progression (rising serum prostate specific antigen, progression of disease on bone scintigraphy, or measurable progressive changes on CT or MR imaging). Patients were imaged with ^{11}C-methionine and ^{18}F-FDG. PET scans were performed with a combination of dynamic acquisition and delayed standard acquisition. Several observations were made in this study. The first was that ^{11}C-labeled methionine had more rapid clearance from the blood than FDG. The serum ^{11}C activity fell to less than half maximum value by 12 minutes in all patients, followed by stabilization or slight increase in serum levels. For FDG, the clearance did not reach half maximum value until 40 to 60 minutes in most patients. For the determination of tumor detection by each of the tracers, a single reference lesion was identified and targeted for evaluation before and after treatment. The degree of uptake in each reference lesion was characterized with a standardized uptake value (SUV). Across all patients, the average SUV_{max} for FDG was 3.47 $\pm$ 0.77, whereas the average SUV_{max} for ^{11}C-methionine was 6.02 $\pm$ 2.1 ($P < .008$).

In a follow-up study,[15] 12 patients with prostate carcinoma and rising PSA levels were prospectively recruited and imaged with ^{11}C-methionine in addition to standard PET imaging with ^{18}F-FDG. In this study, a lesion-by-lesion comparison

was performed using a combination of conventional imaging, follow-up scanning, and biopsy to establish goal standard. In the bones, FDG identified 157 of 325 osseous lesions (48.3%), whereas ^{11}C-methionine PET identified 227 lesions (69.8%). In the abdomen and pelvis, FDG-PET imaging identified 7 of 23 sites of metastatic disease (30.4%), whereas methionine-PET imaging identified 16 of 23 metastatic lesions (69.6%). In total, FDG-PET identified 48% of all sites of metastatic disease, compared with 72.1% for methionine-PET imaging. In this study, the SUVs were higher in sites of metastatic disease imaged with ^{11}C-methionine than with FDG, and this difference in SUV reached statistical significance. There was also a statistical significance in the total number of lesions identified, with more sites of metastatic disease identified on methionine-PET than on FDG-PET. The conclusion of the authors of this study was that ^{11}C-methionine-PET imaging is superior to FDG-PET imaging in the evaluation of patients with prostate cancer.

In a recent study,[16] 20 consecutive patients with elevated serum PSA levels and negative biopsies were imaged using dynamic ^{11}C-methionine PET scanning. Regardless of the findings on methionine-PET scanning, all patients underwent biopsy of the prostate gland. To correlate imaging with biopsy, the findings on methionine-PET scanning were fused with high-resolution MR imaging of the prostate gland, and the combined images were used to direct biopsy by transrectal ultrasound. In cases in which there was focal localization of methionine to portions of the gland, effort was made to target the sites of tracer uptake specifically. Of the 20 patients, 15 had regions of suspicious accumulation of ^{11}C-methionine within the prostate gland. The remaining 5 patients had no areas of suspicious activity. All 5 of the patients with negative methionine-PET scan results had negative prostate biopsy results. Of the 15 patients with focal, suspicious prostatic uptake of the radiotracer, 7 (46.5%) were shown to have malignancy on subsequent biopsy, with a detection rate of 46.7%. In the remaining 8 patients with positive methionine-PET scan results, a histologic diagnosis was made of benign prostatic hypertrophy in 2 and a diagnosis of chronic prostatitis and benign prostatic hypertrophy in 6. The authors acknowledged that biopsies of the methionine-negative group also demonstrated regions of benign prostatic hypertrophy and chronic prostatitis and that the localization of methionine was neither specific nor sensitive for these processes.

The authors concluded that the presence of focal methionine uptake in the prostate gland correlated with a higher likelihood of malignancy diagnosed on subsequent biopsy. They acknowledged, however, that it could not be definitively determined whether the increased detection rate of malignancy after methionine imaging was caused by the affect of image fusion and guidance or the added number of biopsies performed as part of the procedure. This study suggests a possible role for primary evaluation of the prostate gland itself in patients with elevated or rising PSA levels and previous negative biopsy to direct ultrasound-guided needle biopsy of the prostate gland to areas of suspicious activity with the hope of increasing the diagnostic yield of the biopsy procedure.

Additional amino acid tracers have been evaluated using PET imaging, with some preliminary data regarding their use in malignancies of the prostate gland and genitourinary system. One such agent is ^{11}C-labeled C-5-hydroxytryptophan (5-HTP). In a study of 10 patients with hormone-refractory metastatic prostate adenocarcinoma, ^{11}C-5-HTP was evaluated as an imaging agent for detection of metastatic disease.[17] In this preliminary study, all metastatic lesions were visually detected, and the SUV of metastatic lesion was high than in normal bone (2.8 ± 0.60 compared with 1.24 ± 0.46). This difference in SUV was statistically significant. In a subgroup of three patients in this study, imaging was performed before and after therapy. Two patients were treated with strontium-89 for osseous metastatic disease, and one was treated with octreotide. All three patients experienced symptomatic improvement after their therapy. Five lesions in these three patients were imaged with ^{11}C-5-HTP, and in all but one lesion the SUV decreased after treatment.

Imaging with ^{11}C-labeled radiotracers is advantageous because the radiolabeled compound is chemically identical to the nonlabeled compound, with identical biodistribution and clearance. The short half-life of [11]C (20 minutes) limits its general utility and distribution; therefore, there is impetus to develop radiotracers with longer lived isotopes, such as [18]F (110 minutes). One such amino acid derivative that shows promise as an imaging agent for prostate carcinoma is anti-1-amino-3-^{18}F-fluorocyclobutyl-1-carboxylic acid (anti-^{18}F-FACBC). A study performed by Oka and colleagues[18] evaluated anti-^{18}F-FACBC in vitro and in vivo in an animal model. The conclusion of this study was that the contrast of tumor to normal tissue was higher for anti-^{18}F-FACBC than for FDG and that this agent may have the ability to differentiate between prostate carcinoma and benign prostatic hypertrophy in an animal model. A follow-up study was performed in which 15 patients with either newly diagnosed prostate carcinoma or suspected recurrence were imaged with anti-^{18}F-FACBC.[19] In evaluation of the prostate gland itself, the authors noted agreement between visual analysis of anti-^{18}F-FACBC and the results of sextant biopsy (40 of 48 biopsy specimens). The differentiation between sites of malignant biopsy and benign biopsy based on SUV analysis was narrow, however. In general, regions of benign prostate tissue and prostatitis had lower focal uptake than sites of malignancy. Although the primary focus of the study was the prostate gland itself and the correlation of anti-^{18}F-FACBC uptake and primary prostate malignancy, the authors did note that sites of metastatic disease were also visualized by anti-^{18}F-FACBC-PET. A summary of the literature on amino acid tracer imaging of prostate cancer is shown in **Table 1**.

Not all amino acid tracers have been found to be useful in the evaluation of prostate carcinoma, however. There are published reports of amino acid tracers cis-4-^{18}F-fluoro-L-proline[20] and O-(2-^{18}F-fluoroethyl)-L-tyrosine[21] for imaging of solid tumors. Both of these studies included

Table 1
Studies of amino acid PET tracers in prostate cancer

Authors	Year	Tracer	Site of Disease	No. Patients	Sensitivity by Patient (%)	Sensitivity by Lesion (%)
Kälkner et al	1997	^{11}C-5-HTP	Metastatic	10	100	100[a]
Macapinlac et al	1999	^{11}C-Met	Metastatic	10	100	100[a]
Nuñez et al	2002	^{11}C-Met	Metastatic	12	100	72.1
Tóth et al	2005	^{11}C-Met	Primary	20	46.7	NA
Schuster et al	2007	FACBC	Primary/recurrence	15	100	NA

Abbreviations: ^{11}C-5-HTP, ^{11}C-5-hydroxytryptophan; ^{11}C-Met, ^{11}C-methionine; FACBC, anti-1-amino-3-^{18}F-fluorocyclobutane-1-carboxylic acid; NA, not available.
[a] Sensitivity calculated based on index lesions only.

a small number of patients with prostate cancer. In the case of the proline derivative, no significant radiotracer accumulation was seen in prostate carcinoma or in tumors of renal, adrenal, or penile origin. The tyrosine derivative showed some tumor localization in patients with head and neck cancer and breast carcinoma but did not show uptake in the two patients with prostate malignancy.

In summary, preliminary studies suggest that there may be a role for radiolabeled amino acid derivatives in the evaluation of patients with prostate carcinoma. Several studies have demonstrated a potential role for imaging with ^{11}C-methionine PET, and the agent anti-^{18}F-FACBC preliminarily shows promise in evaluation of these patients. In the subpopulation of patients with hormone-refractory prostatic adenocarcinoma, the tryptophan derivative ^{11}C-5-HTP also may have a role as an imaging agent. Further studies on these radiotracers need to be performed to determine their possible role in the clinical evaluation of patients with suspected, newly diagnosed, or recurrent prostate carcinoma.

A significant advantage of imaging with amino acid tracers such as ^{11}C-methionine is the rapid serum clearance and tumor localization followed by a prolonged period of steady tumor retention of the tracer. The timing of imaging is less crucial than with FDG and other tracers in which SUVs can vary over time. With specific regards to the prostate gland, the low urinary excretion of methionine is also a distinct advantage over FDG, in which intense tracer activity in the urinary bladder can mask sites of specific localization to the prostate gland or prostate bed. The most significant disadvantage of PET imaging with methionine is the short half-life of ^{11}C, which limits the practicality of distribution and widespread use.

ANDROGEN RECEPTOR IMAGING

One of the key techniques in early treatment of metastatic prostate carcinoma is androgen withdrawal; most tumors respond initially to this form of therapy.[22–24] Over time, however, tumors tend to alter their biology and become resistant to androgen suppression, progressing in the absence of androgen stimulation. There has been interest in examining androgen receptor activity in patients with metastatic prostate carcinoma in the hopes of not only identifying sites of disease but also predicting response to hormonal-modulation therapies. Early studies demonstrated feasibility of generating positron-labeled androgens.[25] Research showed that it was possible to substitute ^{18}F into key positions in selected androgen molecules, such as

testosterone, 5 alpha-dihydrotestosterone (DHT), 19-NOR-testosterone, and 5 alpha-dihydro-19-NOR-testosterone, and retain an acceptable degree of receptor affinity for the labeled androgen derivative. These early studies identified potential candidates for androgen receptor imaging that could be applied to patients.

A study performed in 2004 examined seven patients with progressive metastatic prostate carcinoma with FDG-PET scanning and 16β-[^{18}F]fluoro-5α-dihydrotestosterone (^{18}F-DHT-PET) scanning.[26] A subset of these patients was also imaged after treatment with hormone suppression. This feasibility study showed rapid tumor localization of the ^{18}F-DHT with prolonged retention on delayed imaging. For detection of disease, ^{18}F-DHT was positive in 46 of the 59 total lesions identified by conventional imaging (bone scanning, CT, or MRI). FDG-PET scanning results were positive in 57 of the 59 lesions. The intensity of uptake in sites of tumor was similar between FDG and ^{18}F-DHT, with and average SUV_{max} of 5.28 for 18F-DHT-PET and an average SUV_{max} of 5.22 for FDG-PET. In the small subset of patients imaged before and after therapy, there was a decrease in ^{18}F-DHT activity after treatment. Most of the malignant lesions in this study were in bone (Fig. 2), but there were also soft tissue sites of disease. ^{18}F-DHT localized to both categories of metastatic disease. Researchers also observed that ^{18}F-DHT showed preferential localization to sites of metastatic disease as compared with normal tissue, despite expression of androgen receptors on a variety of normal cells in the body. A companion article analyzed the biodistribution and radiation dosimetry of ^{18}F-DHT, which demonstrated acceptable levels of radiation exposure at the diagnostic dose ranges.[27]

To demonstrate that the uptake of ^{18}F-DHT is receptor mediated, a study of 20 men with advanced prostate carcinoma was performed before and after the administration of an androgen receptor antagonist (flutamide).[28] In this patient group, PET imaging with ^{18}F-DHT demonstrated abnormal sites of tracer localization in 12 of the 20 patients (sensitivity 63%). In most cases, ^{18}F-DHT confirmed lesions known to exist by conventional imaging techniques. In 5 patients, however, FDHT-PET did detect 17 unsuspected sites of metastatic disease: 14 to lymph node and 3 to bone.

Patients with a positive ^{18}F-DHT scan result received flutamide for 1 day followed by repeat imaging. The mean SUV of ^{18}F-DHT localization decreased from a pretreatment level of 7.0 ± 4.7 to 3.0 ± 1.5, and the tumor-to-muscle ratio decreased from 6.9 + 3.9 to 3.0 ± 1.6, reaching

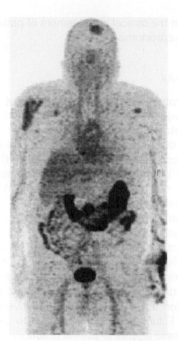

Fig. 2. ^{18}F-FDHT scan of a patient with metastatic prostate cancer. There is uptake in the skull, right upper humerus, and upper thorax at two sites. (*From* Larson SM, Morris M, Gunther I, et al. Tumor localization of 16β-^{18}F-fluoro-5-dihydrotestosterone versus ^{18}F-FDG in patients with progressive, metastatic prostate cancer. J Nucl Med 2004;45(3):369; reprinted by permission of the Society of Nuclear Medicine.)

statistical significance (*P* = .002). By demonstrating this decrease in radiotracer localization after administration of receptor antagonist, it was concluded that the binding and uptake of ^{18}F-DHT in sites of metastatic prostate carcinoma was truly a receptor-mediated process, which supported the hope that this radiotracer may be useful for determining the responsiveness of a patient with metastatic disease to androgen withdrawal therapy. A summary of the literature on F-DHT imaging of prostate cancer is shown in **Table 2**.

The data for PET imaging of prostate cancer with radiolabeled androgen derivatives are not as complete as that for FDG, choline, acetate, and amino acid tracers. The early results are promising, however, for detection and staging of disease and for predicting response to androgen withdrawal. In this sense, imaging of prostate cancer with androgen derivatives matches the new paradigm of PET molecular imaging: personalized therapy based on the genetic and molecular characteristics of a specific patient's tumor, choosing the most appropriate treatment method based on noninvasive probing of tumor biology.

HYPOXIA IMAGING

Tissue hypoxia develops in many solid tumors as a consequence of either rapid tumor growth or the cytotoxic effect of treatment such as chemotherapy or radiotherapy. Diminished blood flow to regions of hypoxia results in impaired delivery of systemic chemotherapies and decreased effectiveness of many compounds,[29,30] and the hypoxic environment incites molecular changes in the tumor cells, which makes them more radioresistant.[31,32] Tissue hypoxia can be assessed invasively with probes, but this is not feasible as a routine clinical tool. The degree of tissue hypoxia within a tumor is typically nonuniform, and multiple measurements would need to be made. There is an interest in noninvasive assessment of tissue hypoxia through imaging in the hopes that such information could be used to predict chemo- and radioresistance and tailor treatment to take these factors—as well as information regarding prognosis[33]—into account.

Various compounds have been developed to assess tissue hypoxia, the most widely used of which are of the nitroimidazole class, which undergo chemical reduction and macromolecule binding in regions of tissue hypoxia. The most widely used imaging compound in this class is ^{18}F-labeled misonidazole, which has been demonstrated to be a safe imaging tracer and has been used to evaluate several types of tumor hypoxia in patients. An early study that examined the use of ^{18}F-labeled misonidazole in quantifying regional

Table 2						
Studies of androgen PET tracers in prostate cancer						
Authors	Year	Tracer	Site of Disease	No. Patients	Sensitivity by Patient (%)	Sensitivity by Lesion (%)
Larson et al	2004	FDHT	Metastatic	7	100	86[a]
Dehdashti et al	2005	FDHT	Metastatic	19	100	78

Abbreviation: FDHT, 16β-[^{18}F]fluoro-5α-dihydrotestosterone.
[a] Calculation excluded two patients with innumerable metastases.

hypoxia enrolled 37 patients with solid tumors, 4 of whom had locally advanced prostate carcinoma treated with radiotherapy.[34] There was wide range of tumor fractional hypoxic volume in these patients with prostate cancer, ranging from 0% to 93.9% (mean, 18.2%). This was one of the first studies showing that hypoxic levels varied within tumor masses, which indicated a possible early need for therapy modulation to overcome the radioresistance resulting from hypoxia. Since that time, however, there have been no clinical studies on the use of hypoxia imaging agents in radiotherapy, chemotherapy, or hormone therapy planning for patients with prostate carcinoma.

Animal-based feasibility studies have demonstrated potential roles for other hypoxic imaging tracers, including ^{18}F-EF5 and copper (II)-diacetyl-bis (N^4-methylthiosemicarbazone). The results of several of these studies[35-38] demonstrated a relationship between disease stage and androgen dependence on levels of tissue hypoxia. The degree of tumor hypoxia was variable in androgen-dependent models, reduced in regressing disease, and significantly increased in androgen independent disease. In the limited studies performed to date, there is a suggestion that imaging of tumor hypoxia may provide relevant information for guiding treatment of patients who have prostate cancer. At this time, however, no conclusions can be made regarding the clinical use of these agents; further studies are needed.

OTHER IMAGING TARGETS

In the arena of oncologic imaging, many other radioisotopes can be imaged with PET. One class of agents is aimed at cellular proliferation with nucleotide analogs. In one study of ^{18}F-18 labeled 1-(2'-deoxy-2'-fluoro-β-D-arabinofuranosyl) thymine (FAMU) in patients with solid tumors, three patients with prostate malignancies were included in the study population.[39] One patient had locally advanced disease arising from the prostate gland, and two had bone metastases in addition to local disease. In two of the patients with in situ prostate tumors, the sites of malignancy were identified with an SUV_{max} of 2.89 and 4.94, respectively. Bone metastases were also identified with good signal to background. A second study with ^{18}F-FAMU in solid tumors also included a small number of patients who had prostate carcinoma.[40] This study demonstrated rapid accumulation of radiotracer within sites of prostate cancer, with little difference in the intensity of tracer uptake when imaged at 5 to 11 minutes compared with 50 to 60 minutes. Despite these suggestive data, no studies have evaluated the role of proliferation imaging

tracers in the clinical management of patients with prostate carcinoma.

SUMMARY

The literature evaluating the imaging of prostate cancer with tracers other than FDG and choline- and acetate-derivatives is limited. The greatest number of articles has examined the role of amino acid tracers, notably ^{11}C-methionine, in the evaluation of patients with prostatic malignancies. A smaller number of studies have looked at steroid-receptor binding, hypoxia, and proliferation as targets for PET imaging of prostate cancer. The conclusion of many of these studies is that there are promising agents apart from FDG, choline/fluorocholine, and acetate/fluoroacetate for the molecular imaging of prostate cancers but that the data are too preliminary to make a recommendation as to their clinical effectiveness and impact. Future studies are needed to define the use of these agents in clinical practice.

REFERENCES

1. American Cancer Society. Surveillance research. Cancer facts and figures 2008. American Cancer Society; 2008. Available at: http://www.Cancer.org. Accessed May 4, 2009.

2. Amis ES, Bigongiari LR, Bluth EI, et al. Pretreatment staging of clinically localized prostate cancer: American College of Radiology. ACR appropriateness criteria. Radiology 2000;215(Suppl):703–8.

3. Lee F, Gray JM, McLeary RD, et al. Transrectal ultrasound in the diagnosis of prostate cancer: location, echogenicity, histopathology, and staging. Prostate 1985;7:117–29.

4. Ohori M, Kattan MW, Utsonomiya T, et al. Do impalpable (T1c) cancers visible on ultrasound differ from those not visible? J Urol 2003;169:964–8.

5. Taoka T, Mayr NA, Lee HJ, et al. Factors influencing visualization of vertebral metastases on MR imaging versus bone scintigraphy. Am J Roentgenol 2001; 176:1525–30.

6. Traill ZC, Telbot D, Golding S, et al. Magnetic resonance imaging versus radionuclide scintigraphy in screening for bone metastases. Clin Radiol 1999; 54:448–51.

7. Wolf JS Jr, Cher M, Dall'era M, et al. The use and accuracy of cross-sectional imaging and fine needle aspiration cytology for detection of pelvic lymph node metastases before radical prostatectomy. J Urol 1995;153:993–9.

8. Jana S, Blaufox MD. Nuclear medicine studies of the prostate, testes, and bladder. Semin Nucl Med 2006;36:51–72.

9. Liu IJ, Zafar MB, Lai YH, et al. Fluorodeoxyglucose positron emission tomography studies in diagnosis and staging of clinically organ-confined prostate cancer. Urology 2001;57:108–11.

10. Oyama N, Akino H, Suzuki Y, et al. FDG PET for evaluating the change of glucose metabolism in prostate cancer after androgen ablation. Nucl Med Commun 2001;22:963–9.

11. Ishiwata W, Ido T, Vaalburg W. Increased amount of D0enantiomer dependent on alkaline concentration in the synthesis of L-[1-^{11}C]methionine. Appl Radiat Isot 1988;39:311–4.

12. Miyazawa H, Arai T, Lio M, et al. PET imaging of non-small-cell lung carcinoma with carbon-11-methionine: relationship between radioactivity uptake and flow cytometric parameters. J Nucl Med 1993;34: 1886–91.

13. Nilsson S, Kalner K, Ginman C, et al. C-11 methionine positron emission tomography in the management of prostate carcinoma. Antibody Immunoconj Radiopharm 1995;8:23–38.

14. Macapinlac HA, Humm JL, Akhurst T, et al. Differential metabolism and pharmacokinetics of L-[1-^{11}C]-methionine and 2- [^{18}F] fluoro-2-deoxy-D-glucose (FDG) in androgen independent prostate cancer. Clin Positron Imaging 1999;2:173–81.

15. Nuñez R, Macapinlac HA, Yeung HWD, et al. Combined ^{18}F-FDG and ^{11}C-methionine PET scans in patients with newly progressive metastatic prostate cancer. J Nucl Med 2002;43:46–55.

16. Tóth G, Lengyel Z, Balkay L, et al. Detection of prostate cancer with ^{11}C-methionine positron emission tomography. J Urol 2005;173:66–9.

17. Kälkner KM, Ginman C, Nilsson S, et al. Positron emission tomography (PET) with ^{11}C-5-hydroxytryptophan (5-HTP) in patients with metastatic hormone-refractory prostatic adenocarcinoma. Nucl Med Biol 1997;24:319–25.

18. Oka S, Hattori R, Kurosaki F, et al. A preliminary study of anti-1-amino-3-^{18}F-fluorocyclobutyl-1-carboxylic acid for the detection of prostate cancer. J Nucl Med 2006;48:46–55.

19. Schuster DM, Votaw JR, Nieh PT, et al. Initial experience with the radiotracer anti-1-amino-3-^{18}F-fluorocyclobutyl-1-carboxylic acid with PET/CT in prostate carcinoma. J Nucl Med 2007;48:56–63.

20. Langen KJ, Börner AR, Müller-Mattheis V, et al. Uptake of cis-4-[^{18}F]fluoro-L-proline in urologic tumors. J Nucl Med 2001;42:752–4.

21. Pauleit D, Stoffels G, Schaden W, et al. PET with O-(2-^{18}F-fluoroethyl)-L-tyrosine in peripheral tumors: first clinical results. J Nucl Med 2005;46: 411–6.

22. Huggins C. The effect of castration, of estrogen and of androgen injections on serum phosphatases in metastatic carcinoma of the prostate: studies on prostate cancer. Cancer Res 1941;1:293–7.

23. Buchanan G, Irvine RA, Coetzee GA, et al. Contribution of the androgen receptor to prostate cancer predisposition and progression. Cancer Metastasis Rev 2001;20:207–23.

24. Loblaw DA, Mendelson DS, Talcott JA, et al. American Society of Clinical Oncology recommendations for the initial hormonal management of androgen-sensitive metastatic, recurrent, or progressive prostate cancer. J Clin Oncol 2004;22:2927–41.

25. Choe YS, Katzenellenbogen JA. Synthesis of C-6 fluoroandrogens: evaluation of ligands for tumor receptor imaging. Steroids 1995;60:414–22.

26. Larson SM, Morris M, Gunther I, et al. Tumor localization of 16β- [^{18}F]fluoro-5α-dihydrotestosterone versus ^{18}F-FDG in patients with progressive, metastatic prostate cancer. J Nucl Med 2004;45: 366–73.

27. Zanzonico PB, Finn R, Penlow KS, et al. PET-based radiation dosimetry in man of ^{18}F-fluorodihydrotestosterone, a new radiotracer for imaging prostate cancer. J Nucl Med 2004;45:1966–71.

28. Dehdashti F, Picus J, Michalski JM, et al. Positron tomographic assessment of androgen receptors in prostatic carcinoma. Eur J Nucl Med Mol Imaging 2005;32:344–50.

29. Kalra R, Jones AM, Kirk J, et al. The effect of hypoxia on acquired drug resistance and response to epidermal growth factor in Chinese hamster lung fibroblasts and human breast-cancer cells in vitro. Int J Cancer 1993;54:650–5.

30. Luk CK, Veinot-Drebot L, Than E, et al. Effect of transient hypoxia on sensitivity to doxorubicin in human and murine cell lines. J Natl Cancer Inst 1990;82:684–92.

31. Coleman CN. Hypoxia in tumors: a paradigm for the approach to biochemical and physiological heterogeneity. J Natl Cancer Inst 1988;80:310–7.

32. Gray LH, Conger AD, Ebert M, et al. The concentration of oxygen dissolved in tissues at the time of irradiation as a factor in radiotherapy. Br J Radiol 1953; 26:638–48.

33. Movsas B, Chapman JD, Hanlon AL, et al. Hypoxic prostate/muscle pO$_2$ ratio predicts for biochemical failure in patients with prostate cancer: preliminary findings. Urology 2002;60:634–9.

34. Rasey JS, Koh W-J, Evans ML, et al. Quantifying regional hypoxia in human tumors with positron emission tomography of ^{18}F-fluoromisonidazole: a pretherapy study of 37 patients. Int J Radiat Oncol Biol Phys 1996;36:417–28.

35. Skov K, Adomat H, Bowden M, et al. Hypoxia in the androgen-dependent Shionogi model for prostate cancer at three stages. Radiat Res 2004;162: 547–53.

36. McNab JA, Yung AC, Kozlowski P. Tissue oxygen tension measurements in the Shionogi model of prostate cancer using 19F MRS and MRI. MAGMA 2004;17:288–95.

37. Yapp DTT, Woo J, Kartono A, et al. Non-invasive evaluation of tumor hypoxia in the Shionogi tumour model fro prostate cancer with ^{18}F-EF5 and positron emission tomography. BJU Int 2007;99:1154–60.

38. Vāvere AL, Lewis JS. Examining the relationship between Cu-ATSM hypoxia selectivity and fatty acid synthetase expression in human prostate cancer cell lines. Nucl Med Biol 2008;35:273–9.

39. Sun H, Sloan A, Manger TH, et al. Imaging DNA synthesis with [^{18}F]FMAU and positron emission tomography in patients with cancer. Eur J Nucl Med Mol Imaging 2005;32:15–22.

40. Tehrani OS, Muzik O, Heilbrun LK, et al. Tumor imaging using 1-(2'-deoxy-2'-fluoro-β-D-arabinofura-nosyl)thymine and PET. J Nucl Med 2007;48:1436–41.

PET and Radiation Therapy Planning and Delivery for Prostate Cancer

Neha Vapiwala, MD[a,*], Alexander Lin, MD[a]

KEYWORDS

- Prostate cancer • PET imaging • CT • MRI
- Radiation treatment planning and delivery
- Image-guided radiation therapy

RADIATION THERAPY FOR PROSTATE CANCER

Prostate cancer is the most common male cancer in the United States, accounting for approximately 25% of incident cases in men, with more than 186,000 cases diagnosed in 2008 alone.[1] The advent of serum prostate-specific antigen (PSA) screening has been linked to a favorable stage shift from distant to more local and regional disease at time of cancer diagnosis, and a coincident decline in cause-specific mortality.[2] The typical staging evaluation after biopsy proof of adenocarcinoma consists of locoregional imaging with pelvic CT and/or MR imaging with or without endorectal coil and distant disease evaluation with bone scintigraphy. Bone scans still may be obtained in patients who are otherwise at low risk for metastatic disease to establish a baseline. Because the number of early-stage cases has continued to increase over the past several decades, so has the role of definitive therapy options. Management recommendations for non-metastatic prostate cancer can vary dramatically but are typically based on patient age, medical co-morbidities, disease characteristics, and geographic location.[3]

The National Comprehensive Cancer Network guidelines list surgery and radiation therapy (RT) as the two accepted initial options for local definitive therapy. Surgical management of prostate cancer involves radical prostatectomy with the conventional retropubic approach or newer laparoscopic- and robotic-assisted approaches. RT is a well-established treatment modality for prostate cancer of all stages in definitive and palliative settings. For clinically localized prostate cancer, the main nonsurgical treatment options are either brachytherapy or external beam RT (EBRT); some institutions advocate use of both RT modalities sequentially.[4] More aggressive and locally advanced disease can be treated primarily with varying combinations and sequences of EBRT, brachytherapy, and androgen deprivation therapy (ADT).[5,6] Brachytherapy comes from the Greek term *brachy*, meaning "short," and is sometimes referred to as sealed source radiotherapy or endocurietherapy.

Brachytherapy as a sole treatment modality for prostate cancer requires appropriate patient selection using relatively strict eligibility guidelines. It can be delivered in two different ways: low-dose rate, permanent seed implantation or high-dose rate, temporary catheter placement. EBRT for prostate cancer also can be delivered in one of two main ways: photons or protons. Photon therapy consists of high-energy megavoltage radiographs produced by linear accelerators, whereas protons are heavy charged particles typically produced in cyclotrons or synchrotrons with notably greater shielding requirements compared with photons.[7] For the purposes of this article, we focus on EBRT for prostate cancer and the

[a] Department of Radiation Oncology, Hospital of the University of Pennsylvania, University of Pennsylvania, 3400 Spruce Street, 2 Donner Building, Philadelphia, PA 19104, USA
* Corresponding author.
E-mail address: vapiwala@xrt.upenn.edu (N. Vapiwala).

PET Clin 4 (2009) 193–207
doi:10.1016/j.cpet.2009.05.005
1556-8598/09/$ – see front matter © 2009 Elsevier Inc. All rights reserved.

role of imaging modalities, including PET, in treatment planning and delivery.

Regardless of the RT modality used, high target doses are essential in the definitive management of prostate cancer, and the dose response with fractionated EBRT is well established.[8–11] Standard fractionation treatment regimens to doses of up to 80 Gy are the standard at many centers. With these high doses, however, comes a higher level of responsibility, and normal tissue protection together with accurate target delineation have been and continue to be the key goals of the radiation oncologist. Even in palliative cases treated to lower total doses, minimizing morbidity from treatment is paramount. Anatomic and functional imaging tools are critical to achieving this favorable therapeutic index and are at the core of most technologic advances in the field of radiation oncology.

ROLE OF TRADITIONAL IMAGING MODALITIES IN PROSTATE RADIATION TREATMENT PLANNING AND DELIVERY
CT-based Planning and Intensity-modulated Radiation Therapy

The introduction and widespread availability of CT in the 1970s and 1980s permitted the development of highly conformal RT delivery. The ability to more accurately and volumetrically define the target and surrounding organs at risk revolutionized the field, and although CT has never been formally tested in a randomized study against the two-dimensional techniques it replaced, it is uniformly and widely accepted as the cornerstone of modern RT planning. A CT simulation is the requisite initial step to the entire planning process, and it entails several important steps: positioning and immobilizing the patient in the planned treatment position; acquiring CT slices throughout the region of interest; immediately identifying the target volume and the isocenter within, where all treatment beams converge; and transfering CT dataset to the treatment-planning software.

The basic steps in standard three-dimensional conformal RT planning involve identifying all target and organs-at-risk structures on axial CT slices, assigning a treatment isocenter within the target volume, and creating a manual "forward-planning" process of trial and error to achieve the ideal combination of beam energy, weight, and angle selections all converging at the isocenter. Treatment plans are ultimately generated and dose-volume histograms evaluated to assess whether target coverage is adequate and organs-at-risk protection acceptable. Unacceptable dose distributions require manual modifications of the beam parameters in a repetitive and relatively time-consuming process. **Fig. 1** demonstrates the steps of structure delineation on the planning CT and dose-volume histogram assessment.

Intensity-modulated RT (IMRT) is essentially the most advanced form of three-dimensional conformal RT and is primarily the result of major innovations in hardware (eg, multi-leaf collimator) and software (eg, inverse planning algorithms). The optimization algorithm is "inverse" in that a dose prescription is specified a priori, and an algorithm is used to work backward to find the dose distribution and corresponding beam parameters that match the desired prescription as closely as possible. Oldham and colleagues[12] were among the first to demonstrate the clinically relevant advantages of inverse planning over forward planning in terms of superior dosimetry and greater efficiency. Although IMRT certainly has limitations and potential disadvantages, the details of which are outside the scope of this article,[13] it is firmly established as the optimal photon-based treatment for prostate cancer. **Fig. 2** demonstrates an example of two approved prostate IMRT plans, with dose color washes representing relative dose distributions throughout the treatment field.

To fully appreciate the fundamental reliance of prostate RT planning on three-dimensional imaging, one should first be familiar with the definitions outlined in the Reports 50 and 62 from the International Commission on Radiation Units and Measurements (ICRU).[14,15] **Fig. 3** depicts these ICRU definitions and helps to visualize the concepts behind them. Accurate delineation of the gross tumor volume naturally requires the most detailed three-dimensional anatomic imaging possible during planning, and MR imaging can provide better definition of the prostate gland from the surrounding nontarget tissues compared with CT. Even with accurate gross tumor volume determination, the use of highly conformal, high-dose fractionated EBRT necessitates and demands precision in the definition of clinical and planning target volumes. In other words, designation of sufficient "safety" margins to account for microscopic disease and for internal and external motion is of tantamount importance and requires real-time imaging during the actual treatments, not just at the time of planning.

MR Imaging

Modern radiation treatment planning for prostate cancer has largely been CT-based. Advances such as IMRT have allowed for the conformal delivery of high doses of radiation to the prostate,

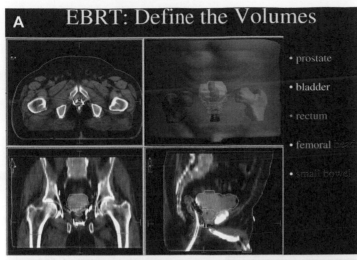

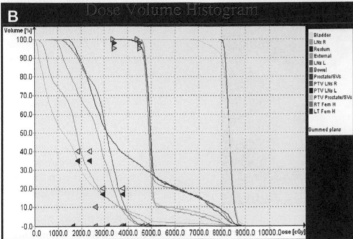

Fig. 1. (A) CT-only–based radiation treatment planning begins with contouring of target and nearby normal organs at risk on axial slices of the planning CT dataset. This treatment is performed by the radiation oncology physician and is based on the specific stage and nature of the patient's disease, together with the anatomic three-dimensional information from the CT. All modern external beam radiation (photons or protons; three-dimensional conformal or intensity-modulated) treatment planning starts with this step. (B) Based on previously mentioned contouring, forward (three-dimensional conformal RT) or inverse (IMRT) planning is performed, and dose-volume histograms are generated. These dose-volume histograms represent the dose distributions to the target and organs at risk and permit assessment of low- and high-dose ranges to ensure that target coverage and organs-at-risk protection are adequate.

with a low risk of severe acute or late toxicity. The ability to visualize and accurately define the prostate and surrounding organs on imaging is important. MR imaging, which offers superior soft tissue contrast and multiplanar image acquisition not available with CT, has an emerging role in radiation treatment planning for prostate cancer.

Differentiating the prostate from the surrounding structures can be difficult on CT, particularly at the prostatic apex, where the boundary between the prostate and the tissues of the urogenital diaphragm can be indistinguishable. Visible adjacent structures are used as a reference to define the position of the apex, with an assumption of a fixed distance of 1.5 cm from the apex to the penile bulb. Later studies showed this distance to vary from 0.6 to 2.3 cm; applying the fixed 1.5-cm rule could lead to inaccurate definition of the apex position.[16] The T2-sequence on MR imaging better demonstrates the internal prostatic anatomy, prostatic margins, extent of tumor, and the boundary between

prostate and the urogenital diaphragm (**Fig. 4**). The higher delineation accuracy obtained by MR imaging has been demonstrated by several studies, which show greater interobserver variation and prostate volume overestimation (from 6.5% to up to 34%) with CT.[17–23] Delivery of highly conformal radiation to a target that is over- or underestimated by CT can negate the benefits of advanced radiation techniques and unnecessarily overdose critical adjacent structures. The increased accuracy and smaller prostate volume obtained with MR imaging leads to improved target coverage and reduced doses to normal structures such as the rectum and penile bulb.[17,24,25]

A previous limitation to the use of MR imaging was the inability to generate digitally reconstructed radiographs for patient positioning, which are calculated from CT Hounsfield units. There are several methods of integrating MR imaging into treatment planning, however. The simplest method is via improved recognition of the prostate

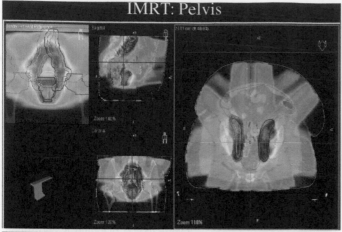

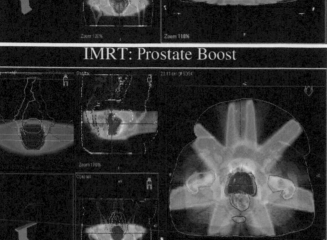

Fig. 2. Color washes show dose distributions of two IMRT treatment plans for a patient with high-risk prostate cancer undergoing definitive radiation. The first plan treats the pelvic nodes (for microscopic disease) and prostate (*top*) and is followed by a second plan for continued treatment of the prostate (*bottom*; ie, boost or conedown). These are both seven-field IMRT plans, with blue, red, and green representing the relatively cold, hot, and intermediate areas, respectively.

and adjacent structures on CT after training in MR imaging anatomy. Another option is to acquire MR images and CT scans and perform side-by-side analysis during contouring of structures. These methods lack full integration of MR imaging data into treatment planning, however, which can only be accomplished with co-registration of CT and MR imaging. It is important to obtain both scans with the patient with an emphasis on reproducibility. Patients are scanned in an immobilized, supine position and are instructed to have an empty rectum and full bladder. Some centers also use daily endorectal balloon for immobilization, which minimizes daily rectal variation and prostate positional variation. This is all done to ensure minimal variation in anatomy at the time of CT and MR imaging scans and daily treatment.

Full integration of MR imaging data into treatment planning requires image registration, which is a potential source of error that can compromise the advantages of MR imaging–based planning. Several complementary methods of registration are available, all with potential sources of error. Registration via mutual information matches

anatomic structures between scans. The prostate is defined as the region of interest, and data sets are cropped to this region. Defining a larger region, such as the pelvis, can help obtain accurate matching of the bony structures of the pelvis but can introduce error in matching of small-volume organs, such as the prostate. Another option for registration involves use of intraprostatic fiducial markers for a seed-to-seed match.[20] Potential sources of error with this technique are from the uncertainty of seed position because of slice thickness artifact. Registration of contours from MR imaging to CT is another option. It requires accurate contouring and, given the significant variability with CT-based contouring, may be prone to errors in the registration.

Improved visualization with MR imaging allows for definition of subtargets within the prostate for additional therapy. T2-weighted MR sequences can identify areas of gross tumor, which has low signal intensity within the high signal intensity background of the normal peripheral zone (**Fig. 5**).[26] Other MR-based techniques, such as dynamic contrast-enhanced MR imaging and MR

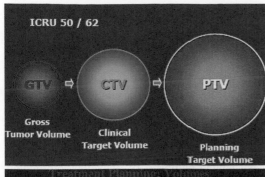

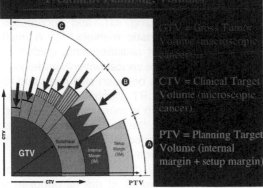

Fig. 3. Two different depictions of the volume definitions for treatment planning, as put forth by the ICRU 50/62.

spectroscopy, can be used to detect intraprostatic lesions, which can be integrated into treatment planning as subtargets for high-dose boost radiation. Recent studies have shown the feasibility of such an approach without adding significant

toxicity to the adjacent surrounding tissue.[27,28] MR imaging also can be used to better define adjacent tissues, because limiting exposure to these tissues is critical to the risk of long-term toxicity. McLaughlin and colleagues[16] used time-of-flight MR imaging angiography to define the internal pudendal artery and other structures critical to erectile function and demonstrated the feasibility of limiting dose to these structures while still maintaining high doses to the prostate. It is expected that as imaging and conformal radiation delivery techniques continue to improve, the concept of boost radiation to areas of high-risk, bulky disease can be accomplished, resulting in improved local control without significant increase in toxicity.

Evolution from Image-guided Radiation Therapy to Adaptive Therapy

Dramatic advances in so-called "on-board imaging" technology are permitting greater precision during actual radiation delivery, thus offering potentially improved therapeutic indices for such patients. Reproducible external immobilization of patients' bony anatomy is typically achieved using skin-based tattoos and a variety of fixation devices.[29] Internal inter- and intrafraction motion have been recognized as the largest contributors to target position uncertainty in tumors otherwise unaffected by respiratory motion, however.[30] Prostate immobilization methods, such as the placement of an endorectal balloon daily throughout the course of therapy, have been reported to decrease positional variability and even

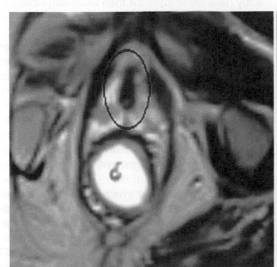

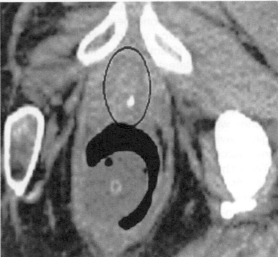

Fig. 4. Genitourinary diaphragm (*defined by red oval*) on axial T2 MR image (*left*), with corresponding CT level (*right*).

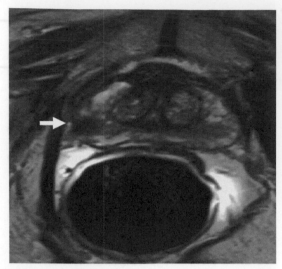

Fig. 5. T2-weighted MR image, axial section. Gross tumor nodule (*arrow*) in the right posterolateral portion of the prostate. Areas of gross disease appear as areas of low signal intensity within the high signal intensity background of the normal peripheral zone.

decrease doses delivered to the rectum.[31–33] The daily reproducibility and reliability of endorectal balloon positioning has been questioned.[34,35]

The assessment and quantification of daily prostate position and interfraction variation over a course of RT have been and continue to be the subject of much concern; when unaccounted for, this internal organ motion is a major cause of target underdosing at the expense of nearby organs at risk. Image-guided RT, an attempt to address this clinical quandary, has evolved over the years from two-dimensional imaging and B-mode acquisition and targeting ultrasound to a diagnostic quality CT-on-rails in the treatment room, to kilovoltage cone beam CT (CBCT), in which the x-ray source and detector are essentially mounted directly on the treatment gantry.[36,37] The latest trends are megavoltage (MV) treatment systems coupled with varying forms of CT technology, such as MV CT (RT machine with an arc of detectors), MV CBCT (RT machine with an on-board electronic portal imaging device), and a CT ring with a rotating MV beam source in lieu of the standard RT machine (ie, TomoTherapy).[38–44]

The leap toward truly adaptive therapy has been made possible through innovations that provide detailed on-board imaging and real-time data on target and organs-at-risk locations to permit any necessary adjustments in the treatment plan and patient positioning, respectively. Examples include the TomoTherapy Highly Integrated Adaptive Radiotherapy (HI-ART) system and the

Calypso 4D Localization System, which is currently FDA-approved only for prostate EBRT.[45] In contrast to image-guided RT, the latter is what one might coin radiofrequency-guided RT. The electromagnetic target localization and tracking system essentially tracks the positions of three transrectally implanted transponders in all three axes relative to treatment isocenter at a frequency of 10 Hz, providing continuous, real-time monitoring of the prostate. Previous studies focusing on intrafraction motion consisted of relatively limited sampling of positional information, from every few seconds to every few minutes, using cine-MR imaging, CT, and fluoroscopic imaging of intraprostatic markers.[46–49] A multi-institutional report of radiofrequency-guided RT in early-stage prostate cancer patients undergoing RT found differences between skin mark and radiofrequency-guided RT alignment of more than 5 mm in vector length in more than 75% of fractions.[50] Qualitatively, the continuous motion was unpredictable and varied from persistent drift to transient rapid movements.

MV CBCT enables direct visualization of soft tissue targets and organs at risk as opposed to orthogonal radiographs of intraprostatic fiducials or ultrasound, which at most provide only target localization. Compared with other direct prostate imaging techniques such as ultrasound, CT-on-rails, and kilovoltage CBCT, MV CBCT offers multiple advantages. It uses conventional radiotherapy equipment (and in this sense even offers an advantage over its close cousin, TomoTherapy), allows for a common isocenter between imaging and treatment, and incorporates imaging dose into treatment planning. MV images inherently have lower contrast than kilovoltage images, however, which may blur prostatic borders, especially at the bladder interface.

Bylund and colleagues[51] examined interfraction prostate motion using MV CBCT and compared their results to other image guidance techniques. Interfraction motion was largest along the antero-posterior axis, which was primarily attributed to systematic bony misalignment. They also reported that interfraction motion of more than 5 mm using MV CBCT was generally similar to or less than that seen with other image-guidance techniques. Less superior-to-inferior motion was observed compared with all other image-guided RT modalities. The authors suggested that decreased visualization of the prostate–bladder interface may possibly lead to an underestimation of superior-to-inferior interfraction motion on MV CBCT imaging. These findings highlight the challenges of lower image contrast for inter- and intrafraction motion and argue for combining various image-guided and radiofrequency-guided RT modalities to acquire complementary information. The design and feasibility of CBCT and electromagnetic target monitoring with proton beam therapy machines are areas of active research, given certain gantry limitations and neutron degradation concerns. Future refinements of high-dose, highly conformal photon and proton-based radiation for prostate cancer undoubtedly will focus on the optimal synergistic use of these various target immobilization, imaging, and tracking techniques in an ultimate effort to achieve the most accurate and precise prostate localization possible before and during treatments.

ROLE OF PET IN PROSTATE RADIATION TREATMENT PLANNING AND DELIVERY

Patients who have prostate cancer comprise just over 10% of the patients enrolled in the National Oncologic PET Registry. This is a remarkable trend considering the relatively small role that PET imaging has played in the management of prostate cancer in past years. Ongoing research efforts seek to further elucidate the use of PET imaging in this patient population. An ultimate goal would be to establish PET as a standard component of the current arsenal of imaging tools used for prostate cancer diagnosis and management, which includes radiotherapy planning and delivery.

Two major obstacles currently stand in the way of widespread incorporation of PET into routine radiation treatment planning. First, to fuse any diagnostic imaging study with the treatment planning CT obtained at time of simulation, the study must have the patient in the exact treatment position as the planning CT. The isocenter coordinates on which the entire treatment plan is based rely heavily on fixed and reproducible patient positioning. In contrast to the couch of a typical PET scanner, the treatment "couch" used for IMRT and proton therapy is actually a relatively uncomfortable, flat, indexed, carbon fiber table. **Fig. 6** represents an example of the misalignment issues that can occur because of small differences in patient alignment and the nature of the imaging couch versus the treatment table. Even if a PET scan could not be directly fused with the planning CT to provide co-registered images, this issue could be somewhat mitigated if PET were to provide high positive and negative predictive values for detection of prostate adenocarcinoma that could reliably guide our treatment planning volumes and fields, especially in terms of nodal basins in which standard imaging modalities are currently limited. To overcome this second obstacle, the development of viable and effective

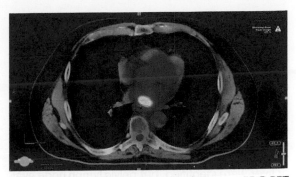

Fig. 6. Example of misregistration between FDG-PET (performed in standard imaging position; target indicated by bright area on scan) and planning CT (performed in radiation treatment position; target indicated by red outline) for a patient with locally advanced adenocarcinoma of the esophagus.

radiotracers for prostate cancer is key. The next section reviews some of these tracers, starting with the most commonly used "gold standard," ^{18}F-fluorodeoxyglucose (FDG).

Fluorodeoxyglucose

FDG is the PET tracer of choice in the oncology world because of its high sensitivity and specificity for evaluation of the presence and extent of malignancy and its relatively long physical half-life and low positron range, which are desirable for imaging. Historically, FDG-PET in prostate cancer management has been considered to be of limited use. Given the inherently heterogeneous nature of the disease, combined with the significant overlap in the metabolic activity of normal prostate tissue, benign prostatic hypertrophy, and frank adenocarcinoma, the value of FDG as a tracer in prostate cancer would seem debatable at best. Others report that certain technical factors may limit the ability to detect clinically significant disease and result in a relatively high rate of false-negative results. For example, filtered-back projection is typically used for image reconstruction, but iterative reconstruction may be preferable for visualization of prostatic activity with FDG-PET.[52] Despite these issues, a growing body of evidence suggests that FDG-PET may be helpful in specific clinical scenarios.[53–68]

In the setting of primary untreated disease, FDG-PET may be used for patients with more aggressive histologic grades (ie, Gleason scores of 8–10) and more locally advanced or metastatic disease. Oyama and colleagues[61,63,64] demonstrated a trend toward higher FDG uptake in tumors with higher Gleason scores and tumors with lymph node and bony metastases. In contrast, the correlation between PSA and FDG uptake by the tumor has not been demonstrated consistently.[64] For detection of nodal and osseous metastases, Shreve and colleagues[67] evaluated 34 patients with biopsy-proven prostate cancer and known or suspected metastatic disease. PET images were read in a blinded manner and compared with the findings from clinical examination, CT, and bone scan. The authors reported sensitivity of FDG-PET for osseous disease of 65%, with a positive predictive value of 98% and estimated standardized uptake value (SUV) of 2.1 to 5.7. Soft tissue metastases to the lymph nodes or liver were identified, but pelvic lymph node evaluation was severely limited because of bladder tracer activity. The authors concluded that FDG-PET can help identify osseous and soft tissue metastases of prostate cancer with a high positive predictive value, but ultimately it is limited and less sensitive than bone scintigraphy in the identification of osseous metastases.[67] There are some potentially provocative findings here, but it is difficult to imagine how FDG-PET in its current state could replace the standard pelvic and bony imaging modalities of CT, MR imaging, and bone scan. It may, at best, enhance these tools.

For recurrent disease after primary local therapy, the data are limited but promising. Chang and colleagues[55] performed FDG-PET imaging followed by pelvic lymph node dissection in patients with rising PSA levels after either radical prostatectomy or RT. All patients had negative whole body bone scans and equivocal findings on pelvic CT. Of the 67% of patients with lymph node positivity, increased FDG uptake was noted in 75% of them at the site of the pathologically positive disease. Four patients had false-negative results, but no patients had a false-positive result on FDG-PET images. The authors reported sensitivity, specificity, accuracy, positive predictive value, and negative predictive value of FDG-PET of 75%, 100%, 83.3%, 100%, and 68%, respectively, for detection of metastatic pelvic lymph nodes.[55] Schoder and colleagues[66] reported that FDG-PET found local or systemic disease in 31% of postprostatectomy patients with PSA relapse; absolute PSA level of 2.4 ng/mL and a PSA velocity of 1.3 ng/mL per year were associated with optimal sensitivity (80%; 71%) and specificity (73%; 77%), respectively.

The clinical relevance of these findings is particularly relevant given that one of the greatest clinical challenges radiation oncologists face is salvage therapy decision making. The inherent dilemma in managing patients with biochemical relapse but without clear radiographic evidence of recurrence using standard imaging modalities is what therapy to offer, when to offer it, and where to direct it in the body. Extraprostatic disease is

found in approximately one third of patients who have prostate cancer after radical prostatectomy alone. Although randomized data clearly demonstrate overall and metastasis-free survival benefits with adjuvant radiation to the prostate bed for pT3N0M0 prostate cancer and/or positive resection margins, many patients are not referred for adjuvant treatment, or if they are referred, they decline it.[69] Fortunately, even in the setting of a rising PSA level postoperatively, there is a reported threefold improvement in prostate cancer-specific survival with salvage prostate bed irradiation compared with no treatment in patients treated within 2 years of biochemical relapse.[70] For postprostatectomy patients, most radiation oncologists ideally recommend salvage radiation before the PSA level reaches 2 ng/mL. Although the current PSA level needed for detection on FDG-PET falls short of ideal, it certainly offers hope for shedding light on an otherwise murky clinical problem.

Finally, for disease that is being actively treated with ADT, either as part of a definitive regimen in combination with EBRT or as a sole modality for noncurative management, FDG-PET may play a role. There is a decrease in FDG uptake after hormonal deprivation in primary prostate cancer sites and metastatic sites. This suppression of glucose use by tumors during ADT may be useful in estimating time to development of androgen-refractory disease, such that treatment regimens and decisions may be individualized based on this prognostic information.[57,62] Of note, an appropriate and effective response to ADT is an undetectable PSA. FDG-PET imaging is not useful in evaluating advanced disease in patients on ADT with undetectable PSA levels. It is of use only if performed before treatment or if the PSA level is rising during treatment (ie, sign of hormone-independent disease).

Perhaps the most important critical advance for FDG-PET that could affect the arena of prostate radiotherapy is its prosperous union with CT in a marriage that mutually benefits both partners. The increasing use of PET/CT in oncology has brought into clinical practice the novel ability to combine three-dimensional anatomic information with metabolic activity, which allows for greater diagnostic accuracy and more precise localization of abnormal structures based not only on size and physical appearance but also on the basis of abnormal metabolic patterns. The interpretation of which metabolic characteristics seen on FDG-PET/CT are normal requires a solid knowledge base of the FDG biodistribution patterns that are typically seen in the organs of interest. Understanding of age-related structural and metabolic changes in certain organs is critical to appropriately distinguish normal physiologic changes from abnormal pathologic variants. For example, it is well established that the normal prostate gland grows significantly over a man's lifetime. Well and colleagues[71] demonstrated that between the second and eighth decades of life, the volume of the prostate gland increased from 23.5 ± 6.2 cm^3 to 47.5 ± 41.6 cm^3; the central gland generally contributes approximately half of this growth and represents an increasing component of the gland with age. This study did not include any data on age-related metabolic changes in the prostate.[71]

In an effort to help establish a "metabolic map" for the normal prostate gland, researchers have analyzed the physiologic metabolic patterns of normal prostate glands using FDG-PET/CT. In one study of 24 men, Wang and colleagues[72] documented an SUV range and mean of 1.6 to 3.4 and 1.9 ± 0.35, respectively. These results confirmed the findings of Jadvar and colleagues,[73] who analyzed more than 140 men with no known clinical, laboratory, or radiographic evidence of prostate pathology and reported a maximum SUV range of 1.1 to 3.7 and population average mean SUV of 1.3 ± 0.4 with this larger sample size. Of note, the authors did not find any statistically significant change in metabolic activity of the normal prostate with increasing age and size, although it is possible that their study of asymptomatic men with "normal" glands may have included subjects with benign prostatic hyperplasia and small unknown deposits of adenocarcinoma.[73] Inherent to any PET study of normal subjects without findings suggestive of prostate cancer is that there is no biopsy-proven disease because there is no biopsy. Another potential confounder is the effect of tumor oxygenation and relative hypoxia on FDG localization in tissue, which can vary based on gland size and tumor histology and extent.[74] Finally, a possible technical limitation is the "feedback" from nearby urinary bladder activity, which generally can be addressed adequately by having the patient void completely just before PET imaging.

Moving from FDG-PET/CT of normal prostate glands to actual prostate cancer, work presented at the recent annual Radiological Society of North America (RSNA) meeting in December 2008 seems promising. Nguyen and colleagues[75] reported on their multi-institutional retrospective study in which 21 patients underwent FDG-PET/CT for staging and 29 patients underwent the same for restaging. PET/CT correctly identified organ-confined and metastatic prostate cancer in 48% of the patients who were imaged for staging purposes. For restaging purposes, biochemical recurrence was defined as PSA level more than 0.4 ng/mL in patients previously treated with prostatectomy and more than 1 ng/mL in patients previously treated with hormonal therapy, RT, or chemotherapy. Of the 29 patients who underwent restaging, 3 were deemed tumor-free, whereas 26 patients had clinically suspicious findings for recurrent disease. PET/CT produced false-negative results in 35% of the suspicious cases but detected disease in the remaining 65% (17 patients). Malignancy was ultimately confirmed in 42% of the patients with suspicious findings. Remarkably, PET/CT also incidentally found second malignancies in 8% of the 50 study patients. Ultimately, however, from the standpoint of EBRT planning and delivery, the need remains for more robust tracers than FDG (see later discussion).

Acetate and Choline

Radiolabeled actetate and choline are frontrunners in the list of prostate cancer PET imaging candidates. A small preliminary study from 2003 comparing ^{11}C-acetate and ^{11}C-choline uptake in prostate cancer found these two tracers to be essentially identical and supported ongoing research of both agents for detection of prostate cancer in local and distant sites.[76] The main issue with ^{11}C as a tracer label is its relatively short half-life ($T_{1/2} = 20$ min), which requires an on-site cyclotron for production. As a result of this need, ^{18}F was subsequently developed; it has a half-life of 110 minutes with a biodistribution that is comparable to that of ^{11}C-choline.[77,78] The main drawback, however, is that ^{18}F-choline does have a markedly greater amount of secretion into the urinary system, which confounds diagnostic quality in the pelvis, the main region of interest for prostate cancer imaging.

As far as localization of prostate cancer, ^{18}F-choline PET/CT does not seem to be ready for prime time, although it may serve a purpose in certain patients with elevated PSA levels but multiple negative prostate biopsy results. In one small study of such a patient population, ^{18}F-choline PET/CT allowed identification of intraprostatic tumor zones in 25% of cases.[79] Similarly, the accuracy of ^{11}C-choline for prostate cancer detection is not well established. ^{11}C-choline PET/CT for lymph node staging in 27 intermediate-risk and 30 high-risk patients who had prostate cancer was compared with two currently used clinical nomograms.[80] All patients ultimately underwent preoperative PET/CT and radical prostatectomy with extended pelvic lymph node dissection. PET/CT showed higher specificity and accuracy than the nomograms; however, the difference was not statistically significantly different. Another study found the sensitivity, specificity, positive predictive value, negative predictive value, and accuracy for ^{11}C-choline to be only 72%, 43%, 64%, 51%, and 60%, respectively; there was no significant correlation between the maximum SUV and PSA levels, Gleason score, or pathologic stage. Some researchers propose that, at most, there may be a role for choline in monitoring response to ADT, because typically there is a decline in SUV after exposure to ADT, just as is seen with FDG.[81]

Returning to the challenging clinical scenario of recurrent disease after prostatectomy, however, there are some compelling data. At the recent annual RSNA meeting, Trampal and colleagues[82] reported on the use of ^{11}C-choline PET/CT for detecting recurrent prostate cancer in 13 patients with increased serum PSA levels (mean, 17.9 ng/mL). Whole-body PET/CT scans were done using ^{11}C-choline; findings were then labeled as positive or negative based on pathologic tracer uptake and later validated with histologic, clinical, or radiologic follow-up data. Overall, ^{11}C-choline picked up disease in 87.5% of patients with a PSA level more than 3 ng/mL and in 40% of the patients with a PSA level less than or equal to 3 ng/mL. Remarkably, based on positive PET/CT findings alone, patients were sent for either local EBRT or systemic therapy (hormonal or chemotherapy) depending on whether they had local or distant recurrence. The investigators remarked that this approach was successful because all patients sent for salvage treatment had subsequent PSA level declines. Of 4 patients with negative PET scan results who were not treated for recurrence, the PSA levels reportedly remain without evidence of disease.

Having said this, it is concerning that biopsies were not performed in all of the cases to confirm either the recurrence or the response to salvage treatment (and corroborate the PSA level declines), because a PSA level decrease in and of itself is not an event specific to cancer therapy. These data are provocative to radiation oncologists, however, because they suggest the existence of locally recurrent prostate cancer cases that can be detected with PET scanning with enough confidence to avoid biopsy. The ability to better distinguish local-only recurrence and oligometastatic disease from widespread distant recurrence has significant implications in medical management.

Perhaps one of the most clinically relevant reports comes from Vees and colleagues,[83] who performed 22 PET/CT studies to assess residual or recurrent tumor after prostatectomy in patients referred for salvage RT. Half of the studies used

[11]C-acetate and the other half used ^{18}F-choline. The key is that all patients had PSA levels of less than 1 ng/mL, with median PSA levels before PET/CT of 0.33 (range 0.08–0.76) ng/mL. In approximately half of the cases, both types of PET/CT studies correctly detected local residual or recurrent disease.[83] Although more research is still needed with these tracers before they can become standard tools, there is a dire need for information to complement studies such as pelvic MR imaging and help further narrow the critical gap between biochemical recurrence and clinical detection. For postprostatectomy patients at high risk of distant relapse but who still have relatively low PSA values, this is the time during which intervention may be life-saving.

Most recently, Rinnab and colleagues[84] reported on ^{11}C-choline PET/CT in 41 patients with a rising PSA level at a mean period of 24 months after prostatectomy. Of note, patients received confirmatory biopsy or surgery as a reference for the PET/CT findings. Six of 12 patients with PSA levels less than 1.5 ng/mL had abnormal uptake on PET/CT, and 4 of these 6 patients (67%) had confirmatory histologic findings. Of 16 patients with PSA levels between 1.5 and 2.5 ng/mL, all of the PET/CT scan results were positive, and 12 of these patients (75%) had positive histologic results. Of 8 patients with PSA levels from 2.5 to 5 ng/mL, PET/CT results were positive, as confirmed by histologic testing in 7 of the 8 (88%). Finally, at PSA levels higher than 5 ng/mL, PET/CT identified disease in all 5 patients, all confirmed by histology. The authors reported an overall sensitivity rate and positive predictive values of ^{11}C-choline PET/CT for detection of recurrence of 93% and 80%, respectively. For patients with PSA levels less than 2.5 ng/mL, the sensitivity rate was 89% with a positive predictive value of 72%.[84]

Thus far we have discussed the issue of local postoperative recurrence in the prostatic bed. Turning our attention to the issue of nodal disease after surgery, Scattoni and colleagues[85] prospectively evaluated the accuracy of integrated ^{11}C-choline PET/CT for diagnosis of lymph node recurrence in 25 patients with rising PSA levels after prostatectomy. Bilateral pelvic or pelvic and retroperitoneal lymph node dissections were performed based on evidence of lymph node metastases on the PET/CT scan in 21 patients and on standard imaging in 4 patients. Of the 4 patients with negative PET/CT and positive MR imaging results, none had nodal metastases. Meanwhile, 19 of the 21 patients (90%) with positive PET/CT result had pathologically positive nodes, with ^{11}C-choline PET/CT sensitivity, specificity, positive predictive value, negative predictive value, and accuracy of 64%, 90%, 86%, 72%, and 77%, respectively. This low negative predictive value reflects the limited capability of ^{11}C-choline PET/CT to pick up disease, and although the overall positive predictive value drops to 70% when the PSA level is less than 2 ng/mL, it offers promise as a guide for treatment decisions.

Rinnab and colleagues[86] also conducted a prospective study to investigate the diagnostic value of ^{11}C-choline PET/CT in 15 patients with rising PSA levels and suspected lymph node metastases. They underwent salvage lymph node dissection for uptake in at least one lymph node. Uptake was seen in nodes along the external and internal and common iliac arteries and in the para-aortic region, with histologic confirmation in 8 of the 15 patients. Although the patient cohort is small, the authors concluded that ^{11}C-choline PET/CT may be useful in this setting. Unfortunately, the clinical benefit of PET/CT and subsequent salvage lymph node dissection was small, with only 1 patient achieving biochemical control.[86]

In conclusion, although studies of PET/CT with these newer tracers have demonstrated small but real successes, we are not yet at the point of establishing a clear role for PET in localization of prostate cancer recurrence. The biggest deterrent is the limited use at clinically meaningful (ie, low) PSA levels.[87,88]

Bombesin

Bombesin, a linear tetradecapeptide, and its related peptide, gastrin-releasing peptide (GRP), can interact with the GRP-receptor (GRP-R) to promote growth of tumor cells.[89–91] The expression of GRP-Rs in prostate cancer has been relatively well documented.[92,93] Bombesin-like peptides have been used as carriers of radionuclides or cytotoxic drugs for the imaging/therapy of tumors that express GRP-Rs.[94–97]

The clinical experience with radiolabeled bombesin analogs for prostate cancer is limited to date. Van de Wiele and colleagues[98] used ^{99m}Tc-labeled bombesin in four patients who had prostate cancer; results showed selective uptake in only one of the four patients. Another study included 10 patients, in whom ^{99m}Tc-bombesin scans were performed.[99] Two of the 10 total patients had benign adenomas; the remaining patients all had prostate cancer. Neither patient with adenoma had tracer uptake, whereas all eight patients who had prostate cancer demonstrated uptake in the prostate. Three patients demonstrated uptake in the first-echelon obturator

nodes. De Vincentis and colleagues[100] studied 14 patients (12 with prostate cancer, 2 with benign adenoma) and performed CT, MR imaging, and ^{99m}Tc scans on all patients. The ^{99m}Tc-bombesin single photon emission CT results were positive in all 12 patients who had cancer, with 4 patients demonstrating uptake in regional lymph nodes. CT and MR imaging demonstrated similar findings in only 3 of the 12 patients.

The role of bombesin-like peptides in the diagnosis of, staging of, and therapy for prostate cancer is an area of active investigation. Although not yet widely used, its potential role in improving staging may help in the selection of patients best suited for radiotherapy or identification of areas amenable for image-guided radiotherapy in the future.

SUMMARY

PET imaging has become an integral component of the diagnosis and management of a substantial number of lymphatic and solid malignancies. Prostate cancer, although one of the most prevalent oncologic entities, is heterogeneous in terms of its behavior and prognosis; therefore it must be so in its treatments as well. Prostate adenocarcinoma has significant physiologic and morphologic overlap with benign and precancerous conditions of the prostate gland, posing a particular challenge in terms of acquiring clinically meaningful metabolic information. One of the greatest dilemmas in prostate cancer remains the need for greater personalization of treatment recommendations based on the true extent of disease, such that patients with extraprostatic, micrometastatic disease can be identified early and managed accordingly. Radiation oncologists specifically would benefit from more precise tailoring of external beam therapy to subclinical sites of disease. These sites currently remain under the level of detection with standard imaging and continue to confound clinicians. Novel PET tracers to complement anatomic data from CT and MR imaging can truly make a difference, and ongoing research holds the greatest promise.

REFERENCES

1. Jemal A, Siegel R, Ward E, et al. Cancer statistics, 2008. CA Cancer J Clin 2008;58(2):71–96.
2. Etzioni R, Tsodikov A, Mariotto A, et al. Quantifying the role of PSA screening in the US prostate cancer mortality decline. Cancer Causes Control 2008; 19(2):175–81.

3. Gregorio DI, Huang L, DeChello LM, et al. Place of residence effect on likelihood of surviving prostate cancer. Ann Epidemiol 2007;17(7):520–4.

4. Dattoli M, Wallner K, True L, et al. Long-term outcomes after treatment with brachytherapy and supplemental conformal radiation for prostate cancer patients having intermediate and high-risk features. Cancer 2007;110(3):551–5.

5. Bolla M, Collette L, Blank L, et al. Long-term results with immediate androgen suppression and external irradiation in patients with locally advanced prostate cancer (an EORTC study): a phase III randomised trial. Lancet 2002; 360(9327):103–6.

6. Hanks GE, Pajak TF, Porter A, et al. Phase III trial of long-term adjuvant androgen deprivation after neo-adjuvant hormonal cytoreduction and radiotherapy in locally advanced carcinoma of the prostate: the Radiation Therapy Oncology Group protocol 92-02. J Clin Oncol 2003;21(21):3972–8.

7. Nakashima H, Nakane Y, Masukawa F, et al. Radiation safety design for the J-PARC project. Radiat Prot Dosimetry 2005;115(1–4):564–8.

8. Dearnaley DP, Sydes MR, Graham JD, et al. Escalated-dose versus standard-dose conformal radiotherapy in prostate cancer: first results from the MRC RT01 randomised controlled trial. Lancet Oncol 2007;8(6):475–87.

9. Kuban DA, Tucker SL, Dong L, et al. Long-term results of the M.D. Anderson randomized dose-escalation trial for prostate cancer. Int J Radiat Oncol Biol Phys 2008;70(1):67–74.

10. Peeters ST, Heemsbergen WD, Koper PC, et al. Dose-response in radiotherapy for localized prostate cancer: results of the Dutch multicenter randomized phase III trial comparing 68 Gy of radiotherapy with 78 Gy. J Clin Oncol 2006; 24(13):1990–6.

11. Zietman AL, DeSilvio ML, Slater JD, et al. Comparison of conventional-dose vs high-dose conformal radiation therapy in clinically localized adenocarcinoma of the prostate: a randomized controlled trial. JAMA 2005;294(10):1233–9.

12. Oldham M, Neal A, Webb S. A comparison of conventional forward planning with inverse planning for 3D conformal radiotherapy of the prostate. Radiother Oncol 1995;35(3):248–62.

13. Lee AK, Frank SJ. Update on radiation therapy in prostate cancer. Hematol Oncol Clin North Am 2006;20(4):857–78.

14. Measurements ICoRUa. Prescribing, recording, and reporting photon beam therapy (report 50). Journal of the ICRU 1993.

15. Measurements ICoRUa. ICRU. Report 62: prescribing, recording and reporting photon beam therapy (supplement to ICRU report 50). Journal of the ICRU 1999.

16. McLaughlin PW, Narayana V, Meirovitz A, et al. Vessel-sparing prostate radiotherapy: dose limitation to critical erectile vascular structures (internal pudendal artery and corpus cavernosum) defined by MRI. Int J Radiat Oncol Biol Phys 2005;61(1):20–31.

17. Debois M, Oyen R, Maes F, et al. The contribution of magnetic resonance imaging to the three-dimensional treatment planning of localized prostate cancer. Int J Radiat Oncol Biol Phys 1999;45(4):857–65.

18. Kagawa K, Lee WR, Schultheiss TE, et al. Initial clinical assessment of CT-MRI image fusion software in localization of the prostate for 3D conformal radiation therapy. Int J Radiat Oncol Biol Phys 1997;38(2):319–25.

19. Khoo VS, Padhani AR, Tanner SF, et al. Comparison of MRI with CT for the radiotherapy planning of prostate cancer: a feasibility study. Br J Radiol 1999;72(858):590–7.

20. Parker CC, Damyanovich A, Haycocks T, et al. Magnetic resonance imaging in the radiation treatment planning of localized prostate cancer using intra-prostatic fiducial markers for computed tomography co-registration. Radiother Oncol 2003;66(2):217–24.

21. Rasch C, Barillot I, Remeijer P, et al. Definition of the prostate in CT and MRI: a multi-observer study. Int J Radiat Oncol Biol Phys 1999;43(1):57–66.

22. Roach M 3rd, Faillace-Akazawa P, Malfatti C, et al. Prostate volumes defined by magnetic resonance imaging and computerized tomographic scans for three-dimensional conformal radiotherapy. Int J Radiat Oncol Biol Phys 1996;35(5):1011–8.

23. Villeirs GM, Van Vaerenbergh K, Vakaet L, et al. Interobserver delineation variation using CT versus combined CT + MRI in intensity-modulated radiotherapy for prostate cancer. Strahlenther Onkol 2005;181(7):424–30.

24. Steenbakkers RJ, Deurloo KE, Nowak PJ, et al. Reduction of dose delivered to the rectum and bulb of the penis using MRI delineation for radiotherapy of the prostate. Int J Radiat Oncol Biol Phys 2003;57(5):1269–79.

25. Yeung AR, Vargas CE, Falchook A, et al. Dose-volume differences for computed tomography and magnetic resonance imaging segmentation and planning for proton prostate cancer therapy. Int J Radiat Oncol Biol Phys 2008;72(5):1426–33.

26. De Meerleer G, Villeirs G, Bral S, et al. The magnetic resonance detected intraprostatic lesion in prostate cancer: planning and delivery of intensity-modulated radiotherapy. Radiother Oncol 2005;75(3):325–33.

27. Pickett B, Vigneault E, Kurhanewicz J, et al. Static field intensity modulation to treat a dominant intraprostatic lesion to 90 Gy compared to seven field 3-dimensional radiotherapy. Int J Radiat Oncol Biol Phys 1999;44(4):921–9.

28. van Lin EN, Futterer JJ, Heijmink SW, et al. IMRT boost dose planning on dominant intraprostatic lesions: gold marker-based three-dimensional fusion of CT with dynamic contrast-enhanced and 1H-spectroscopic MRI. Int J Radiat Oncol Biol Phys 2006;65(1):291–303.

29. Bentel GC, Marks LB, Sherouse GW, et al. The effectiveness of immobilization during prostate irradiation. Int J Radiat Oncol Biol Phys 1995;31(1):143–8.

30. Langen KM, Jones DT. Organ motion and its management. Int J Radiat Oncol Biol Phys 2001; 50(1):265–78.

31. D'Amico AV, Manola J, Loffredo M, et al. A practical method to achieve prostate gland immobilization and target verification for daily treatment. Int J Radiat Oncol Biol Phys 2001;51(5):1431–6.

32. Teh BS, Woo SY, Mai WY, et al. Clinical experience with intensity-modulated radiation therapy (IMRT) for prostate cancer with the use of rectal balloon for prostate immobilization. Med Dosim 2002; 27(2):105–13.

33. Wachter S, Gerstner N, Dorner D, et al. The influence of a rectal balloon tube as internal immobilization device on variations of volumes and dose-volume histograms during treatment course of conformal radiotherapy for prostate cancer. Int J Radiat Oncol Biol Phys 2002;52(1):91–100.

34. Canning CGM, Hung A. Daily verification of prostate motion both with and without a rectal balloon (RB) over the course of treatment. Int J Radiat Oncol Biol Phys 2005;63:S336.

35. van Lin EN, van der Vight LP, Witjes JA, et al. The effect of an endorectal balloon and off-line correction on the interfraction systematic and random prostate position variations: a comparative study. Int J Radiat Oncol Biol Phys 2005;61(1):278–88.

36. Jaffray DA, Siewerdsen JH, Wong JW, et al. Flat-panel cone-beam computed tomography for image-guided radiation therapy. Int J Radiat Oncol Biol Phys 2002;53(5):1337–49.

37. Letourneau D, Martinez AA, Lockman D, et al. Assessment of residual error for online cone-beam CT-guided treatment of prostate cancer patients. Int J Radiat Oncol Biol Phys 2005;62(4): 1239–46.

38. Langen KM, Zhang Y, Andrews RD, et al. Initial experience with megavoltage (MV) CT guidance for daily prostate alignments. Int J Radiat Oncol Biol Phys 2005;62(5):1517–24.

39. Mackie TR, Kapatoes J, Ruchala K, et al. Image guidance for precise conformal radiotherapy. Int J Radiat Oncol Biol Phys 2003;56(1):89–105.

40. Nakagawa K, Aoki Y, Tago M, et al. Megavoltage CT-assisted stereotactic radiosurgery for thoracic tumors: original research in the treatment of thoracic neoplasms. Int J Radiat Oncol Biol Phys 2000;48(2):449–57.

41. Pouliot J, Bani-Hashemi A, Chen J, et al. Low-dose megavoltage cone-beam CT for radiation therapy. Int J Radiat Oncol Biol Phys 2005;61(2):552–60.

42. Ruchala KJ, Olivera GH, Schloesser EA, et al. Megavoltage CT on a tomotherapy system. Phys Med Biol 1999;44(10):2597–621.

43. Seppi EJ, Munro P, Johnsen SW, et al. Megavoltage cone-beam computed tomography using a high-efficiency image receptor. Int J Radiat Oncol Biol Phys 2003;55(3):793–803.

44. Uematsu M, Sonderegger M, Shioda A, et al. Daily positioning accuracy of frameless stereotactic radiation therapy with a fusion of computed tomography and linear accelerator (focal) unit: evaluation of z-axis with a z-marker. Radiother Oncol 1999;50(3):337–9.

45. Welsh JS, Lock M, Harari PM, et al. Clinical implementation of adaptive helical tomotherapy: a unique approach to image-guided intensity modulated radiotherapy. Technol Cancer Res Treat 2006;5(5): 465–79.

46. Aubry JF, Beaulieu L, Girouard LM, et al. Measurements of intrafraction motion and interfraction and intrafraction rotation of prostate by three-dimensional analysis of daily portal imaging with radiopaque markers. Int J Radiat Oncol Biol Phys 2004;60(1):30–9.

47. Britton KR, Takai Y, Mitsuya M, et al. Evaluation of inter- and intrafraction organ motion during intensity modulated radiation therapy (IMRT) for localized prostate cancer measured by a newly developed on-board image-guided system. Radiat Med 2005;23(1):14–24.

48. Ghilezan MJ, Jaffray DA, Siewerdsen JH, et al. Prostate gland motion assessed with cine-magnetic resonance imaging (cine-MRI). Int J Radiat Oncol Biol Phys 2005;62(2):406–17.

49. Mah D, Freedman G, Milestone B, et al. Measurement of intrafractional prostate motion using magnetic resonance imaging. Int J Radiat Oncol Biol Phys 2002;54(2):568–75.

50. Kupelian P, Willoughby T, Mahadevan A, et al. Multi-institutional clinical experience with the Calypso system in localization and continuous, real-time monitoring of the prostate gland during external radiotherapy. Int J Radiat Oncol Biol Phys 2007; 67(4):1088–98.

51. Bylund KC, Bayouth JE, Smith MC, et al. Analysis of interfraction prostate motion using megavoltage cone beam computed tomography. Int J Radiat Oncol Biol Phys 2008;72(3):949–56.

52. Turlakow A, Larson SM, Coakley F, et al. Local detection of prostate cancer by positron emission tomography with 2-fluorodeoxyglucose: comparison of filtered back projection and iterative reconstruction with segmented attenuation correction. Q J Nucl Med 2001;45(3):235–44.

53. Agus DB, Golde DW, Sgouros G, et al. Positron emission tomography of a human prostate cancer xenograft: association of changes in deoxyglucose accumulation with other measures of outcome following androgen withdrawal. Cancer Res 1998; 58(14):3009–14.

54. Bucerius J, Ahmadzadehfar H, Hortling N, et al. Incidental diagnosis of a PSA-negative prostate cancer by 18FDG PET/CT in a patient with hypopharyngeal cancer. Prostate Cancer Prostatic Dis 2007;10(3):307–10.

55. Chang CH, Wu HC, Tsai JJ, et al. Detecting metastatic pelvic lymph nodes by 18F-2-deoxyglucose positron emission tomography in patients with prostate-specific antigen relapse after treatment for localized prostate cancer. Urol Int 2003;70(4):311–5.

56. Jadvar H, Pinski JK, Conti PS. FDG PET in suspected recurrent and metastatic prostate cancer. Oncol Rep 2003;10(5):1485–8.

57. Jadvar H, Xiankui L, Shahinian A, et al. Glucose metabolism of human prostate cancer mouse xenografts. Mol Imaging 2005;4(2):91–7.

58. Larson SM, Morris M, Gunther I, et al. Tumor localization of 16beta-18F-fluoro-5alpha-dihydrotestosterone versus 18F-FDG in patients with progressive, metastatic prostate cancer. J Nucl Med 2004; 45(3):366–73.

59. Morris MJ, Akhurst T, Larson SM, et al. Fluorodeoxyglucose positron emission tomography as an outcome measure for castrate metastatic prostate cancer treated with antimicrotubule chemotherapy. Clin Cancer Res 2005;11(9):3210–6.

60. Morris MJ, Akhurst T, Osman I, et al. Fluorinated deoxyglucose positron emission tomography imaging in progressive metastatic prostate cancer. Urology 2002;59(6):913–8.

61. Oyama N, Akino H, Kanamaru H, et al. [Fluorodeoxyglucose positron emission tomography in diagnosis of untreated prostate cancer]. Nippon Rinsho 1998;56(8):2052–5 [in Japanese].

62. Oyama N, Akino H, Suzuki Y, et al. FDG PET for evaluating the change of glucose metabolism in prostate cancer after androgen ablation. Nucl Med Commun 2001;22(9):963–9.

63. Oyama N, Akino H, Suzuki Y, et al. Prognostic value of 2-deoxy-2-[F-18]fluoro-D-glucose positron emission tomography imaging for patients with prostate cancer. Mol Imaging Biol 2002;4(1):99–104.

64. Oyama N, Akino H, Suzuki Y, et al. The increased accumulation of [18F]fluorodeoxyglucose in untreated prostate cancer. Jpn J Clin Oncol 1999; 29(12):623–9.

65. Oyama N, Kim J, Jones LA, et al. MicroPET assessment of androgenic control of glucose and acetate uptake in the rat prostate and a prostate cancer tumor model. Nucl Med Biol 2002;29(8):783–90.

66. Schoder H, Herrmann K, Gonen M, et al. 2-[18F]fluoro-2-deoxyglucose positron emission tomography for the detection of disease in patients with prostate-specific antigen relapse after radical prostatectomy. Clin Cancer Res 2005;11(13):4761–9.

67. Shreve PD, Grossman HB, Gross MD, et al. Metastatic prostate cancer: initial findings of PET with 2-deoxy-2-[F-18]fluoro-D-glucose. Radiology 1996; 199(3):751–6.

68. Sung J, Espiritu JI, Segall GM, et al. Fluorodeoxyglucose positron emission tomography studies in the diagnosis and staging of clinically advanced prostate cancer. BJU Int 2003;92(1):24–7.

69. Thompson IM, Tangen CM, Paradelo J, et al. Adjuvant radiotherapy for pathological T3N0M0 prostate cancer significantly reduces risk of metastases and improves survival: long-term followup of a randomized clinical trial. J Urol 2009; 181(3):956–62.

70. Trock BJ, Han M, Freedland SJ, et al. Prostate cancer-specific survival following salvage radiotherapy vs observation in men with biochemical recurrence after radical prostatectomy. JAMA 2008;299(23):2760–9.

71. Well D, Yang H, Houseni M, et al. Age-related structural and metabolic changes in the pelvic reproductive end organs. Semin Nucl Med 2007;37(3): 173–84.

72. Wang Y, Chiu E, Rosenberg J, et al. Standardized uptake value atlas: characterization of physiological 2-deoxy-2-[18F]fluoro-D-glucose uptake in normal tissues. Mol Imaging Biol 2007;9(2):83–90.

73. Jadvar H, Ye W, Groshen S, et al. [F-18]-fluorodeoxyglucose PET-CT of the normal prostate gland. Ann Nucl Med 2008;22(9):787–93.

74. Pugachev A, Ruan S, Carlin S, et al. Dependence of FDG uptake on tumor microenvironment. Int J Radiat Oncol Biol Phys 2005;62(2):545–53.

75. Nguyen N. Paper presented at the Radiological Society of North America (RSNA). Chicago (IL), November 30-December 5, 2008.

76. Kotzerke J, Volkmer BG, Glatting G, et al. Intraindividual comparison of [11C]acetate and [11C]choline PET for detection of metastases of prostate cancer. Nuklearmedizin 2003;42(1):25–30.

77. DeGrado TR, Baldwin SW, Wang S, et al. Synthesis and evaluation of (18)F-labeled choline analogs as oncologic PET tracers. J Nucl Med 2001;42(12): 1805–14.

78. Hara T, Kosaka N, Kishi H. Development of (18)F-fluoroethylcholine for cancer imaging with PET: synthesis, biochemistry, and prostate cancer imaging. J Nucl Med 2002;43(2):187–99.

79. Igerc I, Kohlfurst S, Gallowitsch HJ, et al. The value of 18F-choline PET/CT in patients with elevated PSA-level and negative prostate needle biopsy for

localisation of prostate cancer. Eur J Nucl Med Mol Imaging 2008;35(5):976–83.

80. Schiavina R, Scattoni V, Castellucci P, et al. 11C-choline positron emission tomography/computerized tomography for preoperative lymph-node staging in intermediate-risk and high-risk prostate cancer: comparison with clinical staging nomograms. Eur Urol 2008;54(2):392–401.

81. Giovacchini G, Picchio M, Coradeschi E, et al. [(11)C]choline uptake with PET/CT for the initial diagnosis of prostate cancer: relation to PSA levels, tumour stage and anti-androgenic therapy. Eur J Nucl Med Mol Imaging 2008;35(6):1065–73.

82. Trampal C. Paper presented at the Radiological Society of North America (RSNA). Chicago (IL), November 30-December 5, 2008.

83. Vees H, Buchegger F, Albrecht S, et al. 18F-choline and/or 11C-acetate positron emission tomography: detection of residual or progressive subclinical disease at very low prostate-specific antigen values (<1 ng/mL) after radical prostatectomy. BJU Int 2007;99(6):1415–20.

84. Rinnab L, Simon J, Hautmann RE, et al. [(11)C]choline PET/CT in prostate cancer patients with biochemical recurrence after radical prostatectomy. World J Urol 2009; Feb [epub ahead of print].

85. Scattoni V, Picchio M, Suardi N, et al. Detection of lymph-node metastases with integrated [11C]choline PET/CT in patients with PSA failure after radical retropubic prostatectomy: results confirmed by open pelvic-retroperitoneal lymphadenectomy. Eur Urol 2007;52(2):423–9.

86. Rinnab L, Mottaghy FM, Simon J, et al. [11C]Choline PET/CT for targeted salvage lymph node dissection in patients with biochemical recurrence after primary curative therapy for prostate cancer: preliminary results of a prospective study. Urol Int 2008;81(2):191–7.

87. Scher B, Seitz M. PET/CT imaging of recurrent prostate cancer. Eur J Nucl Med Mol Imaging 2008;35(1):5–8.

88. Scher B, Seitz M, Albinger W, et al. Value of 11C-choline PET and PET/CT in patients with suspected prostate cancer. Eur J Nucl Med Mol Imaging 2007; 34(1):45–53.

89. Cuttitta F, Carney DN, Mulshine J, et al. Bombesin-like peptides can function as autocrine growth factors in human small-cell lung cancer. Nature 1985;316(6031):823–6.

90. Rozengurt E. Bombesin stimulation of mitogenesis: specific receptors, signal transduction, and early events. Am Rev Respir Dis 1990;142(6 Pt 2):S11–5.

91. Sunday ME, Kaplan LM, Motoyama E, et al. Gastrin-releasing peptide (mammalian bombesin) gene expression in health and disease. Lab Invest 1988;59(1):5–24.

92. Markwalder R, Reubi JC. Gastrin-releasing peptide receptors in the human prostate: relation to neoplastic transformation. Cancer Res 1999;59(5): 1152–9.

93. Reubi JC, Wenger S, Schmuckli-Maurer J, et al. Bombesin receptor subtypes in human cancers: detection with the universal radioligand (125)I-[D-TYR(6), beta-ALA(11), PHE(13), NLE(14)] bombesin(6-14). Clin Cancer Res 2002;8(4): 1139–46.

94. Reubi JC. Peptide receptors as molecular targets for cancer diagnosis and therapy. Endocr Rev 2003;24(4):389–427.

95. Schally AV, Nagy A. Cancer chemotherapy based on targeting of cytotoxic peptide conjugates to their receptors on tumors. Eur J Endocrinol 1999; 141(1):1–14.

96. Van de Wiele C, Dumont F, van Belle S, et al. Is there a role for agonist gastrin-releasing peptide receptor radioligands in tumour imaging? Nucl Med Commun 2001;22(1):5–15.

97. Van Den Bossche B, Van de Wiele C. Receptor imaging in oncology by means of nuclear medicine: current status. J Clin Oncol 2004;22(17): 3593–607.

98. Van de Wiele C, Dumont F, Dierckx RA, et al. Biodistribution and dosimetry of (99m)Tc-RP527, a gastrin-releasing peptide (GRP) agonist for the visualization of GRP receptor-expressing malignancies. J Nucl Med 2001;42(11):1722–7.

99. Scopinaro F, De Vincentis G, Varvarigou AD, et al. 99mTc-bombesin detects prostate cancer and invasion of pelvic lymph nodes. Eur J Nucl Med Mol Imaging 2003;30(10):1378–82.

100. De Vincentis G, Remediani S, Varvarigou AD, et al. Role of 99mTc-bombesin scan in diagnosis and staging of prostate cancer. Cancer Biother Radiopharm 2004;19(1):81–4.

Index

PET Clin 4 (2009) 209–211
doi:10.1016/S1556-8598(09)00113-8

Moving?

Make sure your subscription moves with you!

To notify us of your new address, find your **Clinics Account Number** (located on your mailing label above your name), and contact customer service at:

Email: journalscustomerservice-usa@elsevier.com

800-654-2452 (subscribers in the U.S. & Canada)
314-447-8871 (subscribers outside of the U.S. & Canada)

Fax number: 314-447-8029

Elsevier Health Sciences Division
Subscription Customer Service
3251 Riverport Lane
Maryland Heights, MO 63043

*To ensure uninterrupted delivery of your subscription, please notify us at least 4 weeks in advance of move.

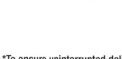
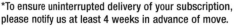

Printed and bound by CPI Group (UK) Ltd, Croydon, CR0 4YY

03/10/2024

01040348-0015